Somber Suffocation

By Morgan Hannaleck

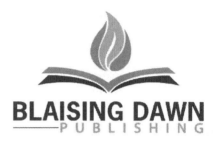

BLAISING DAWN
P U B L I S H I N G

The Heart of the Berkshires, Lenox, MA 01240
www.sombersuffocation.com

Somber Suffocation
Author: Morgan Hannaleck
Editor: Shera Dawn Hunt
Cover Design: Scott Blaise
Publisher: Blaising Dawn Publishing, LLC

ISBN-13: 978-1544107400
ISBN-10: 1544107404

Chapter List

Forward

There are only a few times in our lives when something smacks us in the face and opens us to a world that we may have never known otherwise. I am no exception to this rule; for me that moment was the day I was able to read a story written by a new friend of mine. It was one of the only times in my life that I started and ended a literary work on the same day. Well, except for the days I was being forced to by some over-zealous professor. I was engrossed, emotionally attached, and lost in a world that my wildest dreams could never have possibly fathomed. My eyes carefully followed along word-by-word, sentence-by-sentence; I was reading the words as if the writer was my own daughter and I was finding out for the very first time that she was sick. She wasn't suffering from the flu or seasonal allergies; she had not been diagnosed with cancer. She was sick in a way that I am willing to bet most wouldn't even classify as a sickness, or if they did, it would be one of the last maladies on their list. Eating disorders- far more prevalent than I would've ever imagined and far more secretive than any parent would ever like to admit.

Page by page I entered an unknown world and immediately felt lost. The unknowingness I experienced left me anxious and weary. As a healthcare professional, a nutritionist, and as a father of two daughters, this is a world that I hope to never experience again. Anorexia and bulimia are, however, something that every parent of a teenager, especially a teenage daughter, needs to be aware of as a real threat. It is scary, a mystery to most of us, and, at its core, life threatening. The sad, or better yet, terrifying fact is that Morgan had not contracted this sickness from doctor negligence, a trip to the western plains of Africa, or being sexually irresponsible. No, this very normal and healthy teenage girl caught something that I feel each of us at one point in our lives had come down with...teenage love. I now know that this story runs far deeper than typical teenage love, and at its crux it delved to depths far greater than mere self-esteem issues. Nevertheless, this every day teenage girl was more sick than even her own parents could perceive.

~Dr. Scott Blaise

September 29th, 2016

Prologue

The chiming of my iPhone alarm rudely awakens me like any other Thursday. This Thursday, however, is different. I slowly get out of bed, my legs and back achy and sore due to the heavy deadlifting I had done the day before. As I make my way downstairs my mind begins to wander towards what my birthday breakfast is going to be today.

I can pick up the faint tone of my mom blow-drying her hair coming to a halt as she is disrupted by the sounds of my dog barking at my awakening. She steps out of the bathroom, her dark hair half dry. You would think by age 55 her hair would be graying, but it's not even close.

"Good Morning Sweetie," she began.

She ran her fingers through her short hair while pointing the hairbrush in her other hand towards a brown Dunkin Donuts bag on the table.

"Happy Birthday."

I smile, while peeking into the bag, to discover a single chocolate frosted donut. After all, birthday macros don't count.

I quickly prepared my usual spinach and egg white omelet and threw it on a plate next to my donut. I placed some plain oats in the microwave and smeared a dollop of almond butter on top.. I watched as the richness of the almond butter melted into a syrup-like consistency on top of the oats.

While enjoying my special birthday breakfast, I began to routinely scroll through my Instagram feed. God, I hate this new Instagram update! Rather than showing you photos in chronological order, it displays them in the order of predicted interest, determined by the like photos you are engrossed in the most. The photo itself had no affect on me, but the caption below caught me by surprise. My eyes were immediately drawn to a post by Courtney, my ex boyfriend's new girlfriend. The photo was posted on September 27th, two days ago. It was a picture of her and Sean together, smiling. The caption that followed read: "Happy Three Year Anniversary."

Has it been *that* long since they started dating? Suddenly, it clicked. I can't believe it's been *that* long since I've been sick.

You either say how you feel and completely mess up the situation or you don't say anything and mess up yourself instead. **That's what I had done.**

1
February, 2013

Insecurities

"Okay, step on."

The school nurse is a nice guy: big man, friendly and liked by many. I smile at him and do as I'm told.

It's been about two months since my life kind of just fell apart. I dated Sean for 7 months; exactly 7 months. The day he ended things was our seven-month anniversary.

It sounds like I'm overreacting and all...like it's just one of those silly longer-lasting high school relationships that don't actually mean anything. To me, though, it meant everything. I trusted him. I mean, when Corbin dumped me freshman year, I don't think I left my room for 4 months. I wasn't exactly prepared for that kind of reality; just being dumped and left alone by someone who claimed to love you with everything they're capable of.

Then I met Sean. He's the one who showed me what it was like to love passionately again. He's the one I would live and die for and do it all again still to this day just to make him happy. I can't stop thinking back to the journal I gave him. A part of me wonders if he still looks at it. I mean, I could always ask him. We still talk and all, but everything's a mess at the same time. He let me off so gently on December 28th, 2012. He said he was bored of me, like I was some sort of over-used toy; but he still wanted to talk. He's not sure what he wants, so he still keeps in touch with me and keeps me to the side just in case he figures out I'm what he wants. Just in case.

I'm completely aware of this too...in the back of my mind at least. I like to pretend we still have a chance of getting back together; he still tells me he loves me, so that's a valid reason to keep holding on, right? My friends tell me otherwise, but there has to be a reason why I don't let go. There has to be.

"Okay, all set."

My thoughts are interrupted by the deep voice of the school nurse.

"Thanks," I smile. He had me step on the scale backwards in order to take my height simultaneously, so I didn't get to see either. I wonder what my height and weight is this year. I've always been pretty thin, although I do eat a lot of junk...especially after I got dumped. Ugh. I wish I didn't find so much comfort in chocolate ice cream drenched in hot fudge and whipped cream.

Last year around November, at the doctors, I was 5'4" and 102 lbs. I imagine I'm around the same measures now; it's only been like 3 months.

I leave the nurse's office and go back to class. I guess he doesn't get to tell me what my height and weight is.

"How'd it go?" Amelia asked me as I walked into the locker room.

"Well...I failed the hearing test." I spoke my words out of laughter and with the slightest bit of embarrassment.

All the girls in the locker room cracked up. "Seriously? How!?," Amanda said loudly with a huge smile on her face. I shrugged. "I'm not really sure...Guess I have to take it again in a few weeks."

The girls continued to laugh. I began to change out of my gym clothes, and as I take my shirt off, I'm always sure to suck in my stomach. It's a habit...I've never really been happy with my stomach. I mean, I don't really care THAT much, but when I'm changing in front of people, I'd prefer they don't take a look and see the nachos I had last night. I don't really want to be known as a pig.

I slip on my jeans and as I zip up the zipper, they seem a little snug. It makes me wonder, because these pants are a size 3. I've ranged from a 00 to a 0 pretty much ever since I hit puberty, so wearing a 3 and them being a little tight feels kind of weird. Maybe I should worry a little, maybe eat a little healthier. I'm not really sure if I care enough to do that, though. Eating whatever is sort of comforting...it makes me feel good. It takes away the pain for a little while.

The bell rings and I walk out of the gym towards the bus. On the way out, Amelia catches up with me.

"What are you doing later?," She asks.

"I think I'm hanging with Sean."

She sighs.

"Why do you keep this going?"

"What?" I act confused, as if I don't know what she means. But truthfully, I know exactly what she's referring to. We've been through this too many times as it is. Every time I end up hanging out with Sean, in the moment, we act like nothing has changed between us; like we never broke up, like we never went through any of the difficulties within our relationship that we have. I always end up leaving his house practically on cloud nine, or that's what I pretend to be, at least.

Deep down, my stomach is always twisted into a tight knot knowing that when I leave, he won't be texting me until the next time he's bored. Then the cycle just repeats. I try to figure out what's wrong with him; he reassures me there is still hope of us getting back together and that's why it's fine if we still act like we are dating. Oh, I almost forgot the most important rule of whatever the hell this is…he doesn't tell other girls. Yeah, he brags to his guy friends, but when a girl comes along that he wants to talk to, she has no idea. And when I get upset over it, that's my fault, because we aren't dating in the first place. So I have "no reason to be upset."

And that's why it drives Amelia insane: I can't let go of him, that little bit of hope of us getting back together is what keeps me from walking away. Besides, I'm never going to walk out on him. I promised him that a long time ago. Relationships mean being there for each other, and that's what I'll always do for Sean: a shoulder to cry on at 3 in the morning when having a total breakdown, a person to kiss when feeling lonely, an ear to listen when complaining about life. I can be everything to him if that's what he wants. To me, he's everything.

"You know what. Stop letting him take advantage of you." Amelia's tone became serious and slightly assertive.

"He's not," I immediately reply, somewhat defensively. "We just both still have feelings for each other. It's as simple as that, we aren't ready to move on to other people yet. We're friends."

Ha. Friends.

Amelia rolls her eyes and gets on her bus as I continue walking to mine. I sit in a seat, isolated as usual. I put in my ear buds and drown out the world.

As soon as I'm home, my dog greets me at the door. I say hi and realize how hungry I am. I search around a bit and end up in the freezer, where I take 2 Boston crème toaster strudels and plop them in the toaster. I wait in the kitchen.

"Got any plans tonight?," My dad shouts from the computer room.

"Well I think I'm hanging out with Sean. I'm not entirely sure, he hasn't texted me all day." I feel weird and desperate saying that out loud.

Before my dad could answer, my toaster strudels pop. I take them out of the toaster and use both frosting packets to cover each. I bring the strudels upstairs into my mom and dad's room and take a seat on their bed. As I eat, I stare at my phone. No texts.

I guess I have to text Sean first, like usual. It takes him about an hour to answer and when he does, he's in a bit of a bad mood. I can see that just by the way he responds. Although I don't exactly feel all that welcome, we agree to hang out at his house. I go downstairs.

"Mom, can you bring me to Sean's?"

My mom looks up from the mashed potatoes she's making.

"After dinner."

"When's dinner?" I peek into the oven to see chicken cooking.

"Should be ready in about ten. I'll bring you up after that."

2

February, 2013

*Things Change,
People Change*

This is honestly uncomfortable. It always is at first. I sit on the edge of Sean's bed while he's lying down, messing around on his phone. He finishes up a text and looks up at me.

"So how are you?"

I smile. "Good, how are you?"

"Could be worse, could be better."

"I see." The room is silent.

"Did you hand in your job application?"

I applied at Subway a while ago. I don't really think anything will happen, though. My friend Katie applied when she was with me, so I figured I would join her.

"Yeah...I don't think I'll be getting it though. It was kind of a joke to apply, I didn't have anything better to do."

When I said this, Sean's tone changed. Like, completely changed. He smiled and sat up on his bed.

"Now why would any place be stupid enough to just ignore an application from a girl like you?"

He gently placed his hand on me.

"There's nothing special about me," I laughed. "You, on the other hand..."

I throw myself at him. I tell myself I won't do this every time before I come here. We aren't dating, after all. But I always end up getting weak in the knees just by him smiling at me. Every bit of pain and sadness I have felt throughout the day is slowly taken away through each kiss.

He soothes me. I love him. I still love him. I think I'll always love him.

When he drives me home, the car is silent. He's probably just tired. We get to my house and I thank him for driving me home. I sit there for a moment, waiting for him to kiss me good-bye. He doesn't. I lean towards him and gently kiss him on the lips.

"Bye, Sean. I love   you."

He barely kisses me back, and gives half a smile. I wish his mood was like the way it was earlier.

"Night. Love ya too."

He seems hesitant, but I smile and get out of the car. When I get inside, my mom is always the first to be on my case. "Hi sweetie. How'd it go? What'd you guys do?"

"Just hung out." I always say that. There isn't much else to say.

I go straight upstairs and sit on my bed. A part of me thinks I should be happy, but the pain Sean's desire momentarily soothed has returned. I look over to my phone to see I have no texts and think back to a time when I would get home and have a text from Sean right away. "I love you beautiful girl:)," it would say. But here, now, I've got nothing. I can't remember the last time Sean has called or even made me feel remotely beautiful. When he kisses me, I have to admit I feel pretty good about myself, but it's so short lived. In the end, I know it's not out of love. It's all for him. Always has been.

I lay in bed and open the photo album on my phone. I go to my screenshots folder and scroll back quite a bit until I get to screenshots of conversations. I go to the screenshot of the exact text Sean broke up with me in.

I reread it- again, and again.

You've changed.

I'm honestly bored with us.

I don't feel the same way I did when we first started dating.

I lost feelings for you.

Don't blame yourself.

We need to take a break.

I can't help but blame myself. He can't just tell me I've changed and am so boring that it made him want to end our relationship; and then expect me to not feel like this is all my fault. If it's not mine, then whose is it? I'm the one who changed and I'm the one who messed everything up. There's really no other explanation here.

3
February, 2013
Lent

I hate coming here every week. Actually, scratch that. I hate waking up to come here every week. Ever since I was really little, my mom has made me come to church school every Sunday at 9 am. I never want to be here.

"Okay class," the teacher begins. "As I'm sure you all know, Lent is starting on Wednesday."

Lent. I'm almost positive I gave up soda last year, but it lasted for about 2 weeks until I went to a family party where they had the BEST punch ever. Unfortunately, I have no will power and there was orange soda in it. So basically, Lent last year was a total fail.

"Does anyone here know what they'd like to give up for Lent this year?" The class remained silent.

Truthfully, I don't know what I would want to give up this year. I usually just give up a food that I like, but can easily live without. That kind of ruins the entire purpose of Lent when I do that. Maybe I should try to really participate this year and give up something that's really hard to live without, like chocolate. I literally laugh out loud at the thought of giving up chocolate for Lent. I could never do that.

The teacher turns to me in response to my outburst. "Ah, how about you Morgan? What are you going to give up for lent this year?"

I panic for a moment. Without really thinking that clearly, I tell her: "Every unhealthy food." The entire class turns their attention towards me in amazement.

"Seriously? Wow I give you props...I could NEVER do that," Amanda said in amazement.

"Yeah have fun with that," Amelia snickers.

I just smile and shake my head. Why? Why did I say that? I didn't mean it. I probably said it because I had will power on the brain. That, however, is one thing I have no will power for. There's no way I could just give up everything unhealthy, even if I tried. When I get in the car, I tell my mom about it. We laugh together, but then her tone gets a bit more serious.

"I mean, it's not a bad idea. You never give up anything you actually really, really like for Lent. And your entire class believed you! You should give it a shot." I ponder the idea for a bit. Eh, it's only Sunday. I have a few more days until Lent actually begins to decide.

When I get home, I go straight upstairs to my room. My mom doesn't even comment on the fact that I completely ignored my dog to go upstairs right away, because she knows exactly what I'm headed to do: art. When I was young, like really young, I had dreams of being an artist in the future. As I grew older, school became harder and life became busier. There wasn't much to keep me into art, and I sort of drifted from my interest.

However, when Sean and I were approaching our 5th month anniversary, I had wanted to do something really special for him. Something that came from my heart, something that he could show off to his friends and brag about. It came to me: a portrait. I knew I was rusty, I knew art and I hadn't gotten along in quite a bit. I also knew I could pick up where I left off.

With a solid week of skipping lunch to hang out with the art teacher and A LOT of erasing, I finished my portrait of Sean. I don't want to brag or anything, but I think I did a pretty good job. Unfortunately, the day I gave it to him, he was in a rotten mood, which wasn't out of the ordinary. His bad mood was par for the course; maybe from a tough day at school. Therefore, his reaction wasn't nearly as special or appreciative as I'd hoped it would be. It was more of a fake smile, pretending like I made his day the least bit better. It really hurt, considering how much time and effort I put into making it for him (not to mention the entire week I missed out on lunch!), but the one positive thing I got out of it was that I was hooked on art again.

Anyway, ever since I drew that portrait of Sean, I've been wondering why I ever let go of art for so long. I've learned to fall in love with it all over again.

You've changed.

Right now, I'm working on a painting of Marilyn Monroe. It's what I ran upstairs to work on. I feel like creating art is my only purpose right now; it's the one thing that really centers me, and it's also the one thing Sean still praises me for. I think I'm in love with being appreciated and boosted by him here and there more than art itself. I don't even know. I do know I want to finish this painting, though. I put in my ear buds once again to drown out the world. I grab my brush, dip it in paint and fall into my mental escape.

One thing really does irritate me: when my peaceful mental state is interrupted. My music stops playing due to the playback of my ringtone. I look to my phone to see who could possibly be calling me right now, but I don't recognize the number. It is a number with the same area code as me though, so they have to be from around here. I answer.

"Hello?"

"Hi, may I speak to Morgan please?"

"Speaking."

"Hi! I'm Dale, the owner here at the Adam's Subway. I'm calling in regards to your application; one of my employees here recommended you. I'm sure you can guess it was Mia."

We both laugh. Mia is more of Katie's friend, not so much mine. Mia is really, really tiny. Katie told me she suffered with an eating disorder last year, and now she works at Subway, a lot. Frankly, she's really good at it. I feel like it's her escape, considering everywhere else she goes she is probably monitored over what she eats and how she eats it. Mia could be a manager if she wanted. When she sets her mind to something, there is no stopping her.

"Anyway," Dale continued, "I'd like to set up an interview with you, that is, if you're still interested."

Interested?! Of course I'm still interested! "That'd be great!" I try to balance my tone so I don't sound too excited, but not uninterested, either.

"Awesome. One of our managers, Liz, can interview you around 3 on Monday afternoon. Is that okay?"

A huge smile forms on my face. I forgot I could still smile like this, "I'll be there."

"Looking forward to being in contact with you, Morgan! Liz will see you on Monday." Dale hung up the phone. I immediately dropped my paintbrush and ran downstairs to tell my parents the news.

It's no surprise that when I announce the news, my dad is thrilled. My mom, on the other hand, skips right to the whole "If your grades start to slip..." speech. I act like I've listened to the entire speech, then book it back upstairs to text Sean about the news. I hope he's as proud as I am.

"Great job!" His reply can only form a smile of satisfaction on my face. Great job, Morgan.

I suddenly go into a panic. What if I don't get the job? No great job, Morgan. More like, you fail again, Morgan. I can't let anyone down again. I need this job. I actually forgot I was texting Tim this entire time as well, so I'm sure to let him know the news. As usual, he replies with a well-written response full of considerate advice and encouragement.

I forgot to mention him, Tim. When I was a freshman he would text me every day trying to 'get to know me'. Every. Single. Day. Sometimes I answered, sometimes I didn't. The only time I ever found myself texting him first is when I needed someone to talk with. It's strange that I always went to him for advice rather than any of my other friends, but I think it's because he is so trustworthy. He is also there for me 24/7.

So yeah, we ended up becoming friends over endless amounts of texts, some answered, some unanswered. When Corbin broke up with me, he really helped. He was the best shoulder I could have possibly had to cry on. I did feel bad, though, because I heard a rumor that he really liked me. When I started dating Sean, I heard another rumor that he was devastated. I do feel bad about that, because Tim is a really nice guy and all. However, he's not for me. He's not Sean.

4
February, 2013
You got the job

I swear the only thing that got me through the school day was knowing that I had this interview after school. I didn't tell anyone else about it, in case I don't get the job. I don't exactly have that much faith in myself. I'm wearing a grey sweater, dress pants and flats. My hair is curled and my makeup looks natural yet professional; I feel stupid.

My mom thinks that I should dress up just because I have a job interview. I find this ridiculous, especially because this interview is for Subway. They aren't looking for nice pants or curled hair. They're looking for a signature Subway t-shirt on a body that's ready to work and get dirty doing it. Not what I am.

As my dad drives me, I look in the rear-view mirror of the car and immediately look away. We're in my brother's car, so the mirrors are a bit lower and closer than the ones in my dad's. My face is literally a square. It used to be more heart-shaped, but I swear to God my cheeks filled out and my entire face got fatter. Looking in his mirrors is like a cruel reminder of this... I doubt I'll leave a good impression on whoever is interviewing me. If I were them, I'd laugh at the girl with the fat face and dress pants strolling in for an interview at a sub shop. *I've changed.*

I get out of the car. My dad wishes me luck as I walk towards the door, and I enter. There's only one girl working. She's dressed in yoga pants and a t-shirt that has the subway logo across the front. I'm a bit confused, but I approach her and ask for Liz.

"That's me. You're Morgan?" Her eyes are bright green, masked behind a thick layer of both top and bottom eyeliner. She's surprisingly young, pretty too. It is not exactly what you expect when you think of a manager.

"Yes," I say.

"Alright, come on over." She disappears to the back of the store and returns with a clipboard, headed for one of the tables. I sit.

"So you're 16 correct?"

I smile and reply with a friendly "yes," attempting to leave a good impression on her.

"And you don't play any sports or have any other jobs? Lots of free time?"

I immediately get embarrassed. I hate when people ask me if I play sports and I have to say no. It makes me feel so fat and lazy, like I do nothing with my life. I played tennis freshman year with Claire, but I would hardly count that as exercise. I played soccer up until freshman year and I probably would have continued, but the girls on the team for high school are flat out mean. I'm not that good either, compared to them at least. I wouldn't stand a chance. Plus, the running is intense. I couldn't be that in shape if I tried. When it comes to fitness, I'm pretty lazy.

"No and yes," I reply.

"Alright, well everything looks pretty good then. We can start you on Wednesday."

I immediately get confused. "Wait, so I got the job?"

"Yeah. Your application looks pretty good. You seem friendly, hardworking, have lots of free time...that's pretty much all I'm looking for. Dale will call you with the details about Wednesday. See you then."

42

I smile and thank her. When I get to the car wearing the same smile I left with, my dad immediately knows I have my first job.

5

March, 2013

The BMI System

Spanish begins with the usual whines of Selena. I wonder what it is today.

"It's messed up!" You can tell she's furious.

"You're NOT obese."

"They tried to tell Brittany that she's underweight!"

"Brittany's just small. Didn't she say she ate four hotdogs the day they weighed her too?"

"The BMI system is ridiculous."

My ears perk up at the conversation between my classmates. I turn to Amelia.

"What's wrong with Selena?"

"You know how we got weighed and stuff recently? Well, they sent our parents the results last night and according to Selena's BMI, they're trying to tell her that she's obese and she's pretty pissed about it. I think it's funny."

Amelia isn't too fond of Selena, if that wasn't obvious.

"Wait, we got the results back? Did you see yours?"

"Yeah, didn't you?" Amelia glares over at Selena and dramatically rolls her eyes when she turns back towards mine.

"No... my parents didn't even tell me they sent the results."

"That's weird," Amelia replies.

That's annoying. I feel like everyone has seen their results but me. When I get home, I go straight to my mom. "Did you get mailed results that have to do with my height and weight from the school?"

Mom looks up from her book. "Yes, we got it yesterday."

"Why didn't you tell me?"

She looks a bit guilty, yet confused. "Did I need to? You're healthy. I would tell you if you weren't. I didn't think it mattered."

I'm irritated. "Where is it?"

"Morgan, I don't know. You don't need to see it."

"Where. Is. It?"

She points to a huge pile of papers on the coffee table. Without saying a word, I search through the pile. It takes me a solid five minutes to actually find the paper, and when I do, I bring it upstairs. I don't really feel like talking to my mom right now. I open up the paper to see the tiny arrow on the BMI chart in the "average" section. It's close to approaching underweight, but not there.

This makes me feel oddly...bad I guess. When I was in elementary school, I was always the small one. The one that weighed the least. When we would make a human pyramid in school, I'd always be volunteered to be on top by my peers. I always got full fast as a child. I've always been tiny. So to see I'm "average"...I don't know. It makes me feel like I've gained an unnecessary amount of weight. Its like I've ruined my reputation of being "that small girl." It sucks, because that was one thing about myself that I've always really liked. The only thing I liked, actually.

I look over to my height on the chart and read that I am 5'4", which doesn't surprise me. I figured I was that. When I look over to my weight, my stomach instantly drops: 108 pounds.

You've changed.

When have I EVER weighed that much? The most I have ever weighed was 102 pounds back in November. Gaining 6 pounds in 3 months...that's big for me. That's actually disgusting. No wonder I'm average; I hate feeling average. I feel like there's nothing special about me; I'm not super smart or good at sports, I'm not pretty or funny or sweet. I'm just me. The only different thing about me has been my petite frame, which Sean obviously liked as well at one time...at least that was my thinking back then. No wonder he isn't interested in me anymore.

So, starting right now, there are going to be some changes. I'm going to lose some weight. It does not need to be anything drastic, but I've decided to go with what I told my class about Lent. I'm giving up everything unhealthy. Go hard or go home, right? Not one unhealthy food will enter my mouth throughout the period of Lent this year. That gives me enough time to get down a few pounds by the time Easter comes around. This isn't only a promise to God, but it's a promise to myself.

6
March, 2013
The First Day

When I got to work today, it was not what I had in mind. There's actually a lot more to working at Subway than making subs. There is a whole checklist of things you have to do! You have to get them done by the end of your shift or else you can't leave. Which is extremely inconvenient, what if I had plans right after work? I'm trapped there until I fulfill my responsibilities.

Anyway, Liz showed me the ropes on my first day: the recipes for basic subs, how to refill the bottles of dressing, cleaning tables...basic work. Once she had me settled, Mia trained me from there.

There was quite a lot of work to the training, but I found it difficult to concentrate. All I really did was observe Mia. She gets a lot of work done, and she does it pretty fast as well.. She likes to run around the store a lot while doing so, almost as if she's treating work like it's an intense cardio workout. When you really think about it, it kind of is. Rushing from task to task has to burn a decent amount of calories.

I haven't seen her eat yet, which I guess is what I'm waiting to see. I mean, what do former anorexics eat? Does she eat? She's supposed to be "recovered", so I'd imagine she does. I guess I'm just curious because Mia is the weight I want to be. I bet she's around 100 pounds. That's my goal for now.

So, today at school, I started my diet. I had one egg for breakfast. My mom puts cheese in my eggs. I had a glass of orange juice with that, as I usually do. For lunch, I had some celery and baby carrots, which I dipped in ranch. I brought an apple as well, but didn't end up touching that. It's not as hard to go with less food while I am at school merely because I am distracted all day. I am beginning to discover that after school is what is really tricky.

7
March, 2013
Have a Drink

Tonight, I'm going over to my friend Claire's house. I only have my permit, so my mom drives me over. I feel like Claire is the worst host a friend could ever have. When I get to her house, it's always so dark and empty. Until you go towards the staircase of course, where you can see a faint burst of light coming from the entrance to her room. This is paired with the widest variety of music, wide enough to range from Tim McGraw to Mac Miller.

I greet her dogs and race up to her room, as usual. Today, however, the music is absent.

"...so whatcha doin," I say.

Claire smirked.

"You mentioned earlier that you wanted to do something *out there*, right?"

I thought for a moment. I was texting her earlier that day and *did* say that. I nodded.

"Well," she began, "Do you want to drink?"

My heart skipped a beat. I had never drank before. It's unusual for someone of my age in my grade. Most people here have had their first drinks in eighth grade, stealing their dad's beer or sneaking their mom's tequila.

It's not like I could do that, though. You will not find the slightest drop of alcohol in my house, ever. My dad has been a recovering alcoholic for forty years now. It's pretty self-explanatory why my family is completely against drinking.

Do I really want to be like the other people in my grade? I feel like I should be, like it's time to grow up and be like everyone else. Plus, I don't really care too much about what happens to me, so why not?

I nodded again. Claire's mouth curved ear to ear as she entered her closet. I heard her digging around for a few minutes; when she came out she had a plastic bottle filled to the brim with, of course, what *looked* like water. She took two decently sized glasses and filled each with the liquid.

"Drink it all at once," she said. "You won't like the taste, I'm warning you now; but it's very effective. If you drink it quick, it won't taste as bad."

We meet eye to eye and simultaneously drank our glasses. I nearly gagged at the taste.

"I don't feel any different."

"Give it a minute!"

We sat there in silence for about ten minutes when Claire began to turn her head left to right rapidly.

"Try it!!!!!!!!!!" Out of hesitation, I began to turn my head. With every turn, it was like my head wouldn't be able to stop. I felt as if my head would completely fly off if I turned it with enough force. I became quite dizzy and began to laugh. Claire laughed back.

"Isn't it fun?!" I had never witnessed her eyes being *that* big.

Together, we went downstairs and claimed our own territories throughout her living room. As each minute passed, my vision became more and more unclear. I'm guessing it's been around a half hour since I've been "drunk." Tim keeps texting me; I think he's worried. I honestly can't tell what I'm typing back. I keep attempting to respond with "I'm fine," but I doubt that's what I'm *actually* spelling. My vision sucks.

"Why is Tim texting me and asking if you're alright?" Claire murmured.

"How can you even see your phone?," I questioned.

"Because," she began to explain, "I clearly weigh more than you, making the alcohol affect you much more than it affects me."

"How so?"

"Well, you're a lightweight." A lightweight? I don't feel very lightweight...I actually feel really heavy. Claire made her way over to the bathroom, dragging me along, dizzy and dazed.   She pulled a scale from under her sink.

"Step on it," she commanded. I obeyed and watched as the number slowly settled upon 103 lbs. Claire´s eyes lit up like a Christmas tree.

"Wow, how do you do it?" I didn't understand what she meant. She slurred her words in such a desperate tone; I hardly could even tell she was talking. "Wanna know how I stay low?" she continued. I stumbled into her living room, ignoring both her unclear words and gestures. I sunk into the couch as the entire living room spun around me. Claire crawled into the room as if she was a baby attempting to take her first steps.

"One finger doesn't work anymore annnnnnnnnndd I have to use two now."

"What?" I asked.

"When I stick my fingers down my throat to throw up, one doesn't work anymore so I use two now."

She held her fingers up to her mouth as if she was about to force herself to vomit right here and now in the living room. I grabbed my phone and managed to pull up my video camera. I pressed record, or at least I hope I did.

"Explain exactly what you do," I commanded.

She sighed, as if I was some sort of hassle for asking her to repeat her method. "I take TWO fingers, not ONE now, and STICK it DOWN my THROAT."

"Continue." My voice was firm.

"I keep it there until I throw up."

"Why?" I asked.

"So I won't be fat anymore."

I ended the recording and sprawled out across the couch. From there, the spinning room had nullified into a calm black. My dreams were sober.

8

March, 2013

A New Beginning

The touch of my knees to the cold, hardwood floor gives my entire body a chill that rapidly races up my spine. I feel claustrophobic. My parent's bathroom is so small. I put one ear bud into my right ear and press play. I listen.

"I take TWO fingers, not ONE now, and STICK it DOWN my THROAT...I keep it there until I throw up."

I place two fingers as far as I possibly can directly down my throat. I immediately gag and viciously rip my two fingers out of my mouth. I glare down at them to see a fine coat of saliva dripping onto the floor.

"Okay, let's try this again," I think to myself. I repeat the exact same procedure, removing the fingers and all. Tears form in my eyes. This is *not* as easy as Claire made it seem. One last time, this time I'm much more aggressive with it.

As both of my fingers take a plunge down my throat, I can feel my gag reflex already doing its job. I keep them there. I gag more and more, but keep them there. As I continue to gag, I feel the honey bunches of oats I just ate coming back up. Before I know it, I can taste them. I still keep my fingers there.

The vomit seeped through my fingers and plopped into the toilet from my mouth as I keep my fingers in their place. Two minutes and a toilet full of vomit later, I feel I had thrown up enough. As I rush downstairs to get mouthwash and a bottle of water, my presence has caught my dad's attention.

"Are you coming down with a cold? I heard an awful lot of coughing from you up there!"

My entire face becomes completely flushed.

"I-I don't think I am, just a frog in my throat."

That frog is now in the toilet.

Dear Reader,

The sole purpose of this chapter is to display certain gruesome realities of an eating disorder. These words come from a very unhealthy mind. Know that this is *not* by any means instructions on how to harm yourself- the effects of such actions are purely negative and unsafe.

9

March, 2013

What's a Calorie?

I'm working with Kaylea today. She's really pretty, but she's always complaining about how "fat" she is. To be honest, it gets on my nerves.

"Alright, so Kaylea is outside doing trash and you just need to clean the oven, okay?," said Mia.

"Sounds good. You leaving now?"

Mia glanced over at a bag by the register and picked it up. "Here. These cookies broke, so they're all yours."

I look puzzled. "What about Kaylea?"

Mia grins ear to ear as if I know absolutely nothing.

"Kaylea won't eat those. She *used* to eat four to five per shift, until she saw the calorie content and stopped."

"What's the calorie content?"

"I don't know, like three-hundred and fifty calories or something. See ya later!" Mia punches out of the computer and rushes out of the store, leaving the cookies and me alone.

I look in the bag to see what kinds of cookies were in it. There has to be five or six broken cookies in there, but my eyes fall directly upon three-fourths of a double chocolate chunk cookie, taunting me inside of the bag. I remove it from the bag, originally planning to take one bite. That is until the chocolate chunks had melted in my mouth, sending my taste buds straight to heaven.

In the matter of seconds, the cookie is gone. My stomach growls for more cookies, yet my mind roars just a bit louder for more information. I whip out my phone and open up to Google. I look up "calorie facts" and am completely mind blown.

There are 3,500 calories in a pound.

Soft drinks are an example of empty-calorie foods.

I glare over to my second root beer of the day, because who wouldn't take advantage of unlimited free fountain drinks? *What's an empty calorie?*

They supply the body with calories, but very few nutrients.

2,000 calories is a general estimate of how many calories one should have a day to maintain weight. To lose weight, have 1,500.

How do I keep track of calories?
 MyFitnessPal. I open up the app store in my phone and search for MyFitnessPal. It comes up in the matter of seconds. While it's downloading, Kaylea returns inside from doing the trash.

"Kaylea, do you count calories?"

"Well of course! I've had 500 today." It's 7 o'clock at night.

"How many have you had?" My stomach drops as I shrug my shoulders. I make my way into the hallway, then into the bathroom. I'm **sweating.** Since my first purge, I've done it about once or twice a week.

Now, it's time I do it again. The same conditions as last time, of course. In a panic, I repeat the exact same drill. That cookie wasn't nearly as satisfying the second time.

10
March, 2013
Count Every Bite

Today is my first day using MyFitnessPal. I put in my breakfast after I already ate it, and *now* I know I have a few improvements to make. There were eighty calories in the cheese in my one egg. The cheese isn't even that good. Tomorrow, no cheese... and my orange juice has so many calories; one cup is 110, and I probably had twice that in my large glass!

So, turns out an egg and juice aren't really a small breakfast. When I put in the calorie count for my lunch, I am pleasantly surprised. There are about thirty-five calories for my carrots and about forty for my celery. What doesn't impress me, however, is the amount in my ranch dressing that I dip them in. That dollop of dressing, that small, seemingly insignificant little cup full of dressing, was equivalent to three times the rest of my lunch all together: 225 calories. Clearly I have to decrease my intake now.

I have two Nature's Valley granola bars after school. I intended on having one, but my stomach was making noises louder than I thought possible; I lost a bit of control over my hunger and had two. I'm lucky I stopped there. Unfortunately, two of the granola bars equaled 380 calories-way more than an after school snack should be.

For dinner, my mom made tortellini. I have a very, very small serving, thinking it would be about 100 calories; it was 300. After counting my milk (which I never even *thought* to have calories in it), that brings my entire dinner to around 520 calories. Awesome, and I'm still hungry.

By the end of the day, my total was roughly 1,555 calories. It may be 5 more than my original goal, but it's better than usual, right?

11

March, 2013

Baby Steps

Today, I made those little improvements that I had mentioned yesterday. No cheese or orange juice with breakfast, no ranch with lunch, one granola bar afterschool, purposely not finishing milk with dinner... and I'm *starving*. No joke. I could eat all of Friendly's right now. Somehow my total today is 1,020, which is quite a bit in the first place.

I've been doing research online about weight loss. Some things I've learned:

- Pasta, oil, chips, granola, mostly grains in general are the high calorie, must avoid foods
- Fruits and vegetables are low calorie
- Check out diet foods, such as light wheat bread or canned pineapple sweetened with Splenda
- Don't drink calories-only drink water
- Make everything you do an exercise; whether it is chewing gum or tapping your foot in class, make it an exercise

12

April, 2013

Stay Strong

Today was the first day I've decided to skip a meal completely: dinner. I wasn't planning on it, but now, I can't decide if I'm proud of my decision, or regretful. My stomach is saying regretful.

You see, I was planning to have dinner at Claire's today. She eats a lot later than I do and by 8 o'clock we still haven't had anything, and I have to get home. At home, I tell my mom I ate there. When she asks what, I can feel my face becoming flushed and my inner-liar arises. I immediately reply by saying I had spaghetti.

In bed, I decide to check Vine. Vine is a type of social media where people post very short videos of pointless things-it's kind of funny. At the top of my screen, I see *claire54* has posted a new vine. I tap on it. The vine is a short clip showing bread, then turkey, then cheese and finally mayo. Right before the vine ends, a short snippet of Claire eating the sandwich plays. Right then and there, my stomach rumbles. My mind is set on food. I am in bed, dressed for bed, but not ready for bed. Why couldn't I be ready?

My pajamas are on, I'm both comfortable and tired, but there is this consistent rumble coming from my stomach that is beginning to take over. The growls snap at me as they consume my every thought; it's taking every single bit of willpower I have in me right now not to give in. I have two choices: I can lie in bed and force myself to sleep, or I can get up and eat. I can get skinny or remain fat. I continue on in my bed, heart pounding, thoughts racing and stomach scowling. I don't understand how people do this everyday. How does Mia do it? I want her willpower, her control. I want to be thin.

That night, I eventually fell asleep; and each night, it got a little bit easier. In the past month, I haven't felt as hungry as I should be. I feel as if cutting down on food has cut my stomach down as well, leaving me with a small hole to fill everyday. I'm not even sure if I want to fill that hole.

The less hungry I feel, the less I have to eat, which makes things complicated. I still have to eat, to keep my family and friends off my back, but hiding that is a challenge. The majority of the time, I tell them I eat at work. Which is technically true, I nibble on some of the vegetables there every once in awhile.

Dear Reader,

I want to reiterate, this is not a healthy mindset. I hope from the bottom of my heart that no one repeats any actions I have done; as you continue to read, you discover the life-threatening consequences of these decisions I made.

13
April, 2013
You Still Aren't Enough

I am trying not to be concerned that Sean hasn't texted me in five days, because I haven't lost him, right? We're still together, right? I don't think that's right.

It's wrong of me to think we are together, because I know if someone were to ask
  "How's Morgan?" he would say, "I don't know, she's not my girlfriend." Getting together, even as the "friends" we are, is a secret. It's prohibited territory to speak of us still in any form of relationship. Since technically, we're not in one.

So when I saw on Facebook that an eighth grader posts a status about going to the movies with Sean I am not allowed to be upset, right? Wrong.

I am upset. I am mortified. I call Amelia right away to tell her the news.

"No. Fucking. Way."

"I know."

Amelia sighs loudly into the phone. "Don't talk to him! Seriously! Stop now! This is your chance."

"I'm so upset right now I don't think I will be talking to him for a very long time."

Well, that "very long time" didn't last as long as I had hoped. "Hey Morg," I read on my phone. Is that all he's got? He goes to the movies with another girl, who knows what when on there, and all he can say is "Hey Morg"? I reply with a "Hi."

"I'm sorry."

"Oh no, I hope you guys had a good time. Don't worry about it."

"We didn't do anything. I thought of you the whole time."

I began to loosen up. "Really?"

"Yeah."

You see, that's the problem when you're hooked on someone. You're blinded by them. You believe every word they say, or at least you *want* to. You're scared. I'm scared. Love makes you stupid. I'm scared of losing him. Technically, I already did a while ago. He doesn't make me feel like it, though. When we are together, I feel like I never lost him. I'm pretty sure I'd be completely empty if I did.

That's why I am able to forgive him easily. I don't want to jeopardize the last taste of our relationship that I have. I don't want to be a prisoner, trapped by my own worst experiences and merging them into almost everything I pursue. Holding a grudge may not hurt him, but it's guaranteed to hurt me. I will pay the price of my own self-respect and that is why I don't have any.

14

May, 2013

Are There Calories in Alcohol?

Tonight, Brittany and McKenna and I are all going to our first party. It's at a common party spot in the middle of Cheshire and tell my mom that I'm sleeping over at Brittany's house...because technically, I am.

McKenna's boyfriend, Zach, drives us to the party. That way, all three of us can drink. Zach wouldn't. We have a six pack of Smirnoff's with us, but that's it. We each start off with one. I am nervous about this; not the whole getting drunk at a party thing, because trust me, I want that. I am nervous about the calories.

As we walk up the trail to the party, our shoes and legs get muddy and soaked. My shorts sag off me a bit, more than they used to sag. They're a size two.

"Guys, see the light?" McKenna is testing us on our party knowledge.

"Yes, that's the fire," I respond.

We make our way to the fire, and as we walk in we got looks. Some are dirty, some confused. These looks come from those familiar faces that you have come to know, but haven't actually come to associate with.

"Why are five year olds here?" I hear a mean girl from my school say as we approach the massive group of people. She is glaring at Brittany and McKenna, probably because they're tiny. Not me though. I open up my Smirnoff and became nervous; nervous of whom I will talk to, what I will do tonight.

I see Brittany talking to Kelsey, a junior at our school. They both have wide smiles plastered on their faces, so assuming Kelsey is friendly, I walk over. "Hey guys," I began.

"Hey!" Kelsey is excited to see me. She pointed towards my drink.

"Whatcha got there?"

"Smirnoff."

I decide to make conversation. "What do you have?"

Kelsey looks down at her bottle and smiles widely. "Whipped vodka. It's like regular vodka, but with a sweet twist. Want to try?"

I hesitate. There are no nutrition facts, nothing. However, out of past experience, I know vodka does the trick to get me drunk.

I reach towards the bottle. "Thanks," I smile. "How much?"

"However much you want."

I take one big chug and my face scrunches together as if I had smelt some expired milk. Kelsey was looking at me earnestly, and not wanting to disappoint (and even more not wanting to stay sober), I smile.

"That's awesome," I say. "Mind if I have a little more?"

Kelsey nods and begins to talk to Brittany. While her eyes are off of me, I take three more chugs. If I had to estimate, I'd say it was the equivalent of about four to five shots. I'm running on an empty stomach today, more than usual because I got away without dinner, telling Mom I was eating at Brittany's.

The vodka hits me like a brick wall. I suddenly have the urge to be a lot more social. Screw Sean. There are a ton of guys here. I approach one. "Hey! I love your hair," I say. *Is this my way of flirting..?*

"Thanks!" He replies.

"So," I begin as his face became more and more blurry, "I'm looking to make some new friends tonight. Do you think we can be friends?"

He smiles. "Sure!"

"And friends hug!! Can I have one?"

He smirks and hugs me. I feel wanted. I move on to the next guy, and the next guy, and the next guy. *Hugs, friends, hugs, friends.*

I can feel the eyes of other girls hit me out of spite. Am I loud? Maybe. Am I having fun? I think. The night ends in mooching drinks off of random guys and seeing the vague fire with my intoxicated pupils. I get back to Brittany's house as planned, and pass out on her bed.

15

May, 2013

Am I crazy?

At three in the morning my eyes burst open. I check my phone. Nothing. You never exactly know how crazy you are until you start to care for a person. In my case, a lot more than I should be caring.

Occasionally Sean calls me in the middle of the night. I think it's out of guilt. He's usually having some sort of mental breakdown, and I'm there for him. There have been nights where we have been on the phone for so long that I've only gotten three hours of sleep, but I'd do anything for that boy.

A few days ago, my close friend Cat told me how she heard Sean lied to me about what actually happened at the movies with that 8th grader. Half of the time, I do not have a single clue what to believe. The other half, I know he would not have a problem lying to me.

"Why would you accuse me of that," he barks nastily over the phone.

I immediately feel victimized. "Are you saying it's not true?"

"Yes."

I begin to cry. "Sean, then why would people say that? Why would multiple people tell Cat that? Why is it such a big rumor going around your school?"

"Ok I'm sorry."

"So now it's true?"

"Yes, I was scared to tell you." He hardly sounded sincere. I wanted to throw up.

I hung up.

I don't understand how he can live with himself sometimes. I feel as if he strictly sees life from his perspective, which is why I try not to let my emotions get the best of me in these particular situations. As much as I want to take my not fulfilling his needs as a considerable factor as to why he would continually betray me, I can't help but feel he is slowly revealing his true colors through his actions. I want to give him the benefit of the doubt, like I do with everyone. I want to see the good in people. Yet, he exposes himself unintentionally, and I am definitely paying attention. He only seems to love me when it's convenient for him, and from previous beliefs, that isn't what love is, is it?

16

May, 2013

Take Me Higher

So, long story short, I have forgiven Sean. As usual, I couldn't take not talking to him, and he wasn't about to apologize to me a second time so I would talk to him. Eventually, I ended up apologizing, again. My feelings were overlooked... again.

He invited me over his house today, and as to be expected, I came. My mom dropped me off and we go straight to his room. I don't exactly know how we got on the topic, but for some odd reason, we begin to open up on the subject of weed. Did I forget to mention that?

The majority of the time I'm not with Sean (and probably when I'm with him, who knows), he's high. He hid it from me for a few months, until he finally told me. It started off as a thing he did pretty much every weekend, but now, it's more of a thing he does every day. Today I explored a bit more knowledge of that than I should have; I've learned his habits first hand.

"So," he begins, "do you want to do it?" I've smoked weed about twice in my life. Both times were with a few of my friends. I liked it quite a bit for its calming effect; except for the part that made me hungry, of course.

"Um, sure." I reply.

Sean removes his vape from his closet and a medium-sized black box that disperses a funky skunk-like smell that lingers throughout his room. He set up his vape and he was damn proud of it. He continues to tell me how he paid seventy-five dollars for it and how high it gets you, and he isn't shy about being repetitive over that, either.
   He instructs me on how to use the vape: suck in until you can't breathe, hold it in until your face turns purple, then slowly release.

Being devious, we put a movie on his huge television in his room, in order to make sure his mom, who was upstairs, knew we weren't up to any sort of mischief. After about seven long, slow hits, Sean admits he can't do anymore. "I'll stop too," I say. I figure if he does this on the regular, and I weigh a significant amount less than him, I should be good too. I don't exactly feel much different, until suddenly, the movie is repeating itself.

By that, I mean the image of the movie on the screen looks like some sort of never-ending tunnel. It just keeps *repeating, and repeating and repeating*. Whenever Sean tries to talk, his mouth doesn't match up with his words. He becomes cold and ruthless, and every time I try to get closer to him, he acts unattracted to me, and pushes me away.

We both lay down on his bed, where in my mind, everything about my life begins to re-play. I see myself as a five-year-old, playing with Claire in daycare and coloring with washable markers until my little heart was satisfied. I see myself in third grade, being left out of my friend group, but never standing up for myself on how mistreated I was. I see myself in middle school, trying to fit in, trying to be cool, trying to look like I was having the best time of my life. I see myself on my first day of high school, walking around the school as if it was Christmas morning, thinking the next four years would be the best ones of my life. I see myself losing every last bit of innocence

I had, one scenario at a time. I see my happiness fade away as I grew. I see my happiness fade away as I shrunk. "Morgan," I hear.

"MORGAN."

I jump. I think I was asleep, but I can't be sure of that. My mouth feels like someone has put a vacuum to it. "I'm really...thirsty."

Sean hands me a Capri Sun and grumbles. "I gave this to you twenty minutes ago."

I remember him handing it to me, and throwing it to the side. I thought there would be no possible way I can put any of that into my body, but I settle on having one sip. It takes me awhile to get the straw inside of the pouch, and I can feel Sean's fierce glares shooting at me and causing tension to arise in the room. I take one sip. It was the best thing I have ever tasted in my entire life. As it partially quenches my thirst and travels slowly down my throat, the juice feels like a cool tropical wave rushing throughout my entire body.

Making me fat.

Expanding my thighs.

Hurting me.

The next thing I know, Sean's face is an inch away from mine. He kisses me. To take action would mean I would have to know what's going on, but I don't.

I don't have the energy to do anything here. Every word is misunderstood and every sight is distorted. I can only remember his lips to mine, then, everything fading to nothing. Now, I'm in his car.

"Are you sure you're okay to drive?"

Sean's firm tone takes a toll on my stomach. "Yes. I'm **fine.**"

I feel as if any minute, he will take a sudden stop on the side of the road and throw me out of the car. When I arrive at my house, I walk through the door, immediately told my mom I am not feeling well, and stumble upstairs. I fall asleep.

17
May 28th, 2013
One Year

So, I've hit the goal I want to be. I am 100 pounds. It's weird, though. I don't really look much different at all. It's not nearly as satisfying as I thought it would be. I've come to realize that my "goal" isn't what I've really wanted.

I want more.

Is it just me, or do the days go by slower? This lifestyle lengthens time, causing every minute of both hunger and lack of energy to drag on with the most spontaneous kicks and life-sucking twists.

Today would be Sean and my one-year, if we were still *officially* together; I reserve my entire night for him and only him. I spend my afternoon with Claire, working on our history project. As we walk to the door, I turn to her.

"Do you want anything to eat?"

Claire smirks. "Yes. Let's be bad." The controlled, powerful me would have disagreed instantly. I would've said no to the sugar, the fat, the sodium and the calories: the reversed progress.

The weak part of me, however, says yes. Her invitation to binge has intrigued me.   We grab chips, cookies, cupcakes, crackers, brownies... everything. You name it, we take it. We bring our stash upstairs and immediately begin to indulge; I forgot how delectable food can taste.

When you deprive yourself, it really hits you when you finally eat. It hits both of us hard. I glare over at Claire. A beast has unleashed inside of her, a beast that likes cupcakes and potato chips. She looks as if she hasn't eaten in months. Do I look like that?

I put down my fourth cupcake and decide enough is enough. "I'll be right back. I'm not feeling so good." I race downstairs into the bathroom and begin the ritual. Fingers better be clean, because they're going deep, deep down.

The water in the toilet bowl splashed as the colorful remains of cupcakes, chips, and chocolate plop within it. The smell of the toilet bowl, that close and personal, has become an ordinary scent to me. I take a shot of mouthwash as fast as I possibly can and swish it vastly and vigorously.   I rush back upstairs, and put on the pouty look for Claire.

"...you ok?"

"Yeah. I threw up, and now I feel better."

Claire looks suspicious. "That was random."

I had hoped to hide the discomforted look in my eyes, unfortunately my stealthy actions become more apparent by the minute.

"Let's get back to the project."

As the afternoon progresses, Claire knows her time is soon up. She gathers her things. "My dad's coming in five," she announces.

"Okay."

"So," she begins, "what do you think you and Sean are going to do tonight?"

I smile. "Honestly, I don't know. I've talked about it a lot more than he has. He doesn't seem all that excited."

I hear a faint beep coming from the front of my house and turn my cheek.

"Your dad's here."

Claire grabs her backpack and makes her way out of the door. "See ya tomorrow. Good luck."

I grasped onto my phone to check my messages. None. I text him.

"Hey," he responds almost immediately.

"Are we still doing something today?" I stood by my phone for at least ten minutes, counting on a quick reply.

"Maybe."

Maybe? All I get is a maybe? It's been an entire year, our one year; something that used to light up our eyes and give us both the chills when we thought about it, and now it's nearly nothing to him. I don't reply for a while, until the clock hits six; now I feel as if I've been wasting my night.

"Don't mean to be a bother, but do you know if we're doing something or not?"

A good amount of time has passed, when my phone finally buzzes around six-thirty.

"I don't think so."

I look at myself in the mirror and sit down. I had been getting ready to see him since

Claire had left; I've been doing my hair, makeup, outfit and all to perfection.   I tell him it is alright and that maybe we could do something later in the week. I threw on some sweatpants and lay in bed, scrolling through Instagram.

I see that one of his friends has posted a photo with him, his guy friend, and two other girls.   The girl that posted it was a friend of his that he admitted to like a few years ago, and believed was very beautiful. I look at all of them, posing for the picture. He seems content without me. I place my phone on the floor and bury my face into my pillow.

After about five minutes of staining my light blue pillow in both mascara and tears, I storm out of the room. I step on the scale and watch the red line slowly make it's way up to ninety-six pounds. Although down in weight, I am still furious. Lucky for me, I don't eat my feelings anymore; I starve them.

18

May, 2013

My Shift Is Over

Today, Brittany and I are walking on the bike trail. We just had lunch, well I should say she had lunch, I had some lettuce. Obviously it was my idea to walk off the calories. While walking, my phone rings.

"Hello?"

"Hey Morgan, it's Kayla from Subway."
Kayla was another manager.

"Hi Kayla."

"We need you to come into work for 2." It's 1:30.

"I'm not scheduled today."

"You're on call."

"Yes and Mia *called* me and told me I don't have to come in, so I made plans."

My plans were to go to the mall with Sean. He asked me! I jumped on his offer. He only has to return something quickly, but this will be the first time he's taken me out in public in over six months.

"Well that isn't the case anymore. See you at 2."

I begin to get angry. "I can't."

"Morgan. Stop arguing and get here."

"No! This isn't fair!"

"Come into work for your shift, Morgan."

I hesitated for a moment, then snapped. "I quit."

"What?"

"I'm done."

"You're quitting?"

"Yup. Have a good day."

"Morgan, wai-"

I immediately hang up and am reluctant to speak due to the shock of my impulsive decision. I can't say I would've made such a big deal about working if I wasn't going out in public with Sean again, even if it was for like five minutes. Oddly enough, my biggest concern turns out to be how I am going to get away with avoiding dinner now; I usually work from 4-10:30 PM, so work was the perfect excuse, and now I have nothing. I guess I'll just have to step up my game.

19

June, 2013

Maine

Earlier this year my mom had planned a trip to Maine. She said I could bring a friend, and considering my brother decided to take his girlfriend Meg, I took her up on the suggestion and invited Claire.

Once the day of leaving has approached us, we pick up both of the girls and proceed with a long car ride ahead of us. After arriving at the hotel, my mom suggests we go to the beach. This is the moment I've been waiting for, to be able to put on a bathing suit and take pictures in it, finally feeling thin. I flourish off of knowing that posting a photo in a bikini will get me a like from Sean, even if he only misses my body and not my heart.

I put on my blue bandeau bikini top, because this way it's harder to tell I don't have boobs anymore. The bottoms are saggy in the back, but they never used to be. I can't weigh myself for the next four days here because I don't have access to a scale, but my weight before I left was 89 lbs. I've been dropping weight steadily as my habits have become consistent; less binging and purging, more starvation.

I don't realize how exhausting walking through sand is until I googled how many calories it generally burns per hour; that explains things. When Claire and I decide to get into the water I notice her staring at me, for a while too. We prance around in the water, take pictures and talk. Claire and I have no boundaries or filters on what we can say to each other, so I am not shocked when I finally come to realize why she has been staring at me.

"You look like a corpse," she blurted out.

In a way, those words came off to me as one of the most genuine compliments someone has ever given me. I feel empowered. Like I was up to Sean's standards again. Like I was thin, determined and worthy. Like I was almost beautiful.

Claire walks *very* fast, almost too fast, like she is still trying to lose weight. She probably is. I didn't mind, although it is difficult to keep up with her. I basically get 6-7 hours of power walking in for the next four days. We walk around the beach, where I drift away from the shore so I can walk in the sand. We walk laps around the amusement park, walk to restaurants to meet up with my parents and swim too. I can burn a lot of calories and keep busy so I don't have to constantly think about how hungry I really am. We go out to eat three times a day, and every single day I get egg whites and watermelon for breakfast, a half sized portion of a chicken salad (light on the chicken, no cheese, dressing or croutons) for lunch and dinner.

I weigh myself the minute I get home from Maine, where the scale says 83 pounds. I turned vacation into a part of my weight loss quest and feel very content with that.

20

June, 2013

Choices

A few weeks after Maine, Sean starts to make comments about how skinny I am looking. At first I thought they were compliments, but they turn out to be just the opposite. He told his mom about my issues and she says she is worried about me, saying I don't look healthy anymore.

At first, I thought he told his mom about my issues because he was concerned about me, too. Then, as I progressively discover little things he has done with other girls while we were "together" (and lying about it), I soon come to realize that he doesn't have a care in the world about what I am doing to myself. People suspect that I am getting thinner and thinner as a result of how he is treating me, and he knows that. So pretending to care seems like the right choice, right?

I begin to wake up in the middle of the night from multiple intense, vivid nightmares. Most of them involve opening a fridge to find every single one of my favorite foods. In some of the nightmares, I cave in and eat it all. In others, I don't. I still don't know which one is worse. I wake up multiple times a night from hunger pains as well. I wake up hungry for breakfast, wanting breakfast, needing breakfast, but scared for breakfast.

I wake up checking my phone, too. I check for texts from Sean, missed calls from Sean. Usually there is nothing. All together, I wake up around 7-8 times per night. It might actually be easier to say I sleep a few hours each night, but it's okay. Lying awake will burn more calories.

In life, you can make choices, but sometimes choices can make you. There may come a point where you can't decide which is which; today is that day for me.

I find myself crying, sobbing actually; I call my mom into my room.

"Mom," I begin. She sees the tears form, once again, in my eyes.

"Honey, what's wrong?"

I reach under a blanket that is lying around my room only to reveal the bathroom scale to my mother. She glares at it, and her unhinged mind boggles at the tears welling up within my eyes.

"That's where the bathroom scale went!" As her eyes look back into mine, I know there is something amiss about this situation.

I decide I am going to let the scale itself do all of the explaining. I emit a long exhale and take a step on top of it. The scale settles on eighty-two.

"Oh honey," my mom begins, "that scale probably isn't right."

I pull up ten pictures on my phone, all of the same scale; yet with each picture, the number descended a bit more every time. My mom gawks at the photos as a confused expression makes its way upon her face.

"I don't get it," she says.

"Mom, I've been starving myself. I originally wanted to lose a little weight, but only to a degree. Now, I'm getting a little worried I won't be able to stop." She hesitates.

"I felt like something odd was going on with you," she hedges.

Although the confession isn't something she could have anticipated, her expression remains entirely calm. The calmness isn't quite out of disregarding my problem, but more out of denial; like nothing is serious, like I am going to be okay.

Forcing a smile back on her face, she soothes me. "But we can fix this. I'll help you."

Momentarily, she does make me feel like I am going to be okay. However, becoming worried about something I was just praising myself for is slightly alarming. When did my accomplishment become a complication? I just want to be able to stop whenever I feel like it; what shakes me up is the suspicion that I can't.

Dear Reader,

You may think, if in a similar situation, you would be able to control such a thing-know you cannot and no one is "special" when it comes to eating disorders. They are out of your control, no matter what. The disease takes over, **not you**.

21

July, 2013

The Health Scare

My mom hasn't really had much to say to me, ever since I admitted my little secret. All I've really gotten are nods of the head when I pick up something to eat and a stare here and there at my legs. Nothing seems very significant right now. Tonight with Brittany, things are different. I've had a sharp on and off pain in my stomach for a few days now, and it is progressing out of my control tonight.

"Ow!"

"What's wrong?"

Brittany and I are in my room, cleaning through old clothes that I want to get rid of; most of them are too big. "There's searing pain in my stomach."

Brittany's eyes wander throughout my room and slowly brought their way back to mine.

"Do you want me to go home so you can rest?"

I shake my head. This will pass. After about twenty minutes, the pain escalates from a pinch to a punch. I am lying on the ground, unable to move. Brittany brings my mom upstairs, who is on the phone with my doctor.

117

"Honey, it's too late to make you an appointment tonight," she begins, "but there's a spot for you at 7 A.M., bright and early. Do you need something more urgent? Is it that bad?"

I remain on the floor. I can suck it up for a night if I go right to sleep. I almost forget Brittany is even here, until she spoke up.

"Well, it's getting late," she manages to squeak out while quickly gathering her things together, "so my dad probably wants me home. Feel better Morg."

I smile at Brittany as she makes her way out of my door.

In the morning, I devour my eighty-calorie yogurt cup and go straight to the hospital; the pain isn't as severe as yesterday, mainly because I actually found the strength in me to move. The nurses do their usual routine: have me pee in a cup, weigh me, take my temperature, and get my heart rate and blood pressure. Then, the doctor makes her way in.

"Hey Morgan," she sighs, "What's going on?"

I explain the sharp pain keeping me up at night.

"Well, for starters, I'm very concerned about your weight. You've gone down twenty-seven pounds since I last saw you, which was only about six months ago. What's up with that?"

"I-" I begin to choke. I suddenly feel so vulnerable.

"You know Morgan, if you were to get a cold right now, I don't think your body would be able to fight it off. That's how weak you are."

"I'm scared of being fat," I blurt out.

She smiles, as if she is satisfied for getting me to speak.

"Your heart rate is relatively low, but it's currently still stable. I'm going to need you to come in tomorrow morning for some blood tests. Have you ever considered therapy?"

"No."

"I have a great woman I can recommend to you. I'll go talk to your mom." Now, everyone is in on it.

22

July, 2013

Can You Pass Your Drug Test, Miss Morgan?

Shortly after my little brawl with the manager of Subway, I decide to apply to the Big Y, my local grocery store. My brother has worked there for the past three years, and having no problems with it so far, I figure I would give it a shot. I didn't expect anything out of this one application until I am sitting in front of Martha, the woman who runs the show here at the Big Y, telling me that I got the job. My eyes lit up to the best of their ability, as they have been lifeless for a few months now.

"Okay Morgan," Martha starts off as she plops a boatload of paperwork into my open arms, "You need to report to Pittsfield within the next twenty-four hours in order to take a quick drug test before we get you started here. You're just going to have to pee in a cup, nothing special. Will that be okay?"

My stomach drops. Sean. I've smoked with Sean, *a lot of smoke.*

I nod quickly and squirm out of the room like a squirrel after a nut. I dial Brittany's number without any hesitation.

"Hello?"

"Brittany! Your brother smokes and got a job at Target, right? How did he pass his drug test?"

"Drive to the drug store and get some cranberry supplements. Be at my house in ten. And don't stop drinking water."

I did what she asked and reported to her house. We treat this like an operation. I am down almost four liters of water by eight o'clock that night. The drug test is for eight in the morning. I hardly sleep that night. I am up, peeing and drinking, drinking and peeing.

The morning of the drug test has me shaking with nerves. As my brother pulls into the parking lot of where I will be tested, I just finish my fourth water bottle of the morning. I did everything that was asked of me during the test, and all I have left to do is wait.

23
August, 2013
Junior Year

Summer flies by. Each day, I begin to care less and less. I drink more (plain vodka, of course) whenever I have the opportunity. I'm a text away from Sean whenever he needs me. I become his temporary girlfriend; he may even care less than me. At least this way, I can still feel a slight connection to him. This way, I still am able to hear his voice and see his face. I can still look at him and fantasize over what we once had. Any time I can see him, I will take.

I stay with him so he won't have to face his problems alone; whether it is the little, everyday stresses or something bigger. I can be there for him, even though I truly know he doesn't want me there. I chose him over and over again every single day, because I am hopelessly in love with him; and even when I mean nothing to him, I can't make these feelings go away. I can't tell my mind to do something my heart isn't ready for. I never knew how much it could hurt, to be physically sitting next to the boy you love, but not having been mentally with them for a year.

My parents begin to get scared. Other people make comments about my skeptical eating behaviors, and as they observe my body shrink and my true colors fade, they start threatening me. Every once in awhile, they'd make me step on the scale in front of them. Then came the threats-*we're going to send you away to treatment, Morgan.*

Everything I did became an exercise-on top of the 5-6 miles I would run about every other day. I end up slowly gaining a little weight, from my lowest weight to about 93 lbs.-just to keep my parents off my back. I sure as hell miss being my lowest weight, but at least this way I can still be thin and less likely to pass out in front of them. Although I am probably still near my deathbed, I was on even thinner ice when I was 82 pounds-an unpredictable weight.

I end up passing my drug test and getting the job at Big Y. The shifts are short, but they drag on forever. Old ladies accuse me of partying too much due to my lifeless nature and the drained look on my face. Silly customers, I'm actually just dying. My days begin consisting of school, running, work, sleep, waking up, sleep, waking up, sleep, waking up, sleep, waking up, repeat. It is miserable.

24
August, 2013
He Stopped Saying
Goodnight, So I
Stopped Sleeping.

He cares about partying more than he will ever care about you, Morgan are the distraught words tucked in the back of my mind that my frontal lobe refuses to accept.

  I'm on fire; I'm a burning flame, all of the time, for him and only him. He simply uses me as his lighter. For the parties. The smoking.

I'm constantly ready to burst with words that are unsure to me. I see mountains in his eyes, mountains of hope for not only him, but also for us. I don't think he has even seen a single hill in mine. I speak trembling words, and it astonishes me that he is never concerned that my entire being is as unsteady as my sentences. It takes me far too long to perceive that he isn't what I need him to be, and I never can be what he wants me to be. These type of thoughts haunt me in my darkest hours, hours like today.

There it is, the release from these thoughts: the gallon of ice cream, taunting me with it's tasty looks inside of the freezer. "*Indulge,*" it whispers slowly. I can only imagine the ice cold, sugary sensation of both chocolate and guilt rushing down my throat. Maybe I'm wrong, though; it's been so long. After all of this time, I may have just forgotten what ice cream actually tastes like.

Without thinking, and in a demonic panic, I take it out of the freezer. It's freezing touch creates a chill throughout my entire body as it races down my spine. I may be freezing, but at least I'm thin. Stick thin. A fine, exquisite layer of frost might as well form on the surface of my skin before I ever gain a single ounce of weight. Before I know it, I am a completely different person. It is halfway gone and I am continuing to shovel through the rocky-road paradise. I decide to add hot fudge, then whipped cream. Then Oreos, and soon enough I delicately dip the Oreos into a large glass of ice-cold, full fat milk.

Then comes the bread. Going against my thirty-five calorie whole wheat bread is a skinny girl's sin; it's like going against everything I could ever stand for in the past year and a half, but I do it anyways. Drowning my full-sized white bread in both peanut butter and bananas, I gobble that down too. "*Eat me*," they all whisper, hovering around and haunting me with every possible glance I can take.

I'm so desperate here. Ninety-three pounds. It was eighty-two pounds merely a month ago, I don't see how *this* isn't enough: Enough for the doctors, enough for my family, enough for my body, enough for a life. I don't see why I can't remain this weight for the rest of my existence. What's the big deal anyway, why does something as simple and unimportant as *my* personal body weight result in such controversy between every single person involved in *my* life? It's *my* life. I can't get sent away. I won't get sent away. I'm beyond sick of the threats and the constant, head-pounding stress.

Out comes the cheesecake. I wonder if the hot fudge tastes good on that too? Eating and eating, will I ever get full? It's like when I start, I can't stop. This is exactly why I'd rather just not eat in the first place, which I'll be sure to resort back to first thing in the morning, even more intensified than most days due to this little episode.

I race up to my room to grab my stash of laxatives. The box says two, but the thought of fat actually storing in my body causes me to cringe, so I take six. I *need* to get rid of this food. I *need* to remain empty. Everything about me *needs* to be nothing but pure, painful, advancing emptiness. Maybe the laxatives aren't enough to empty myself here. With my stomach full and my mind racing, I make my way over to the bathroom.

I'm sure it won't taste nearly as good the second time.

25
August, 2013

Disposable

It's funny, how quickly you can transition from one end of the spectrum to the other. How kissing someone, touching someone, or even just talking to someone, all things that could signify a passionate bond, ultimately become nothing but a way to pass the time. Being in love with him **was** enchanting. Profusely, day after day, time after time, seeing Sean grows more and more hollow. The value had diminished the day we stopped saying "I love you" whenever we saw each other, like it was no longer necessary, like it was no longer felt. I am drawn to the damage. Eventually, whenever I'm with him, I just check out of my body and wait. Every time, I am not there; I become his possession. I become disposable.

26

September, 2013

In the Blink of an Eye, He's Gone.

Sean has been acting odd and distant lately-more than usual, that is. He invites me over today, and something is much different about today as compared to any other. I usually care about how I look around him-actually no-I usually make sure to look the best I can for him. Today, however, I don't care. I throw on the nearest pair of pants I can find, along with a sweater to match. They both sag off of my body, but I don't care about that, either.

I brush through my hair and relent to style it. I make my way to his house.
Our habitual routine has dulled into nothing. I feel no emotion anymore. Every time I kissed, touched, or even looked into his eyes, I gave a tiny piece of my heart away. Eventually, there was nothing left. Lying face-up on his bed, glancing back and forth between him and my hipbones, everything feels futile. It's frustrating. What an inner turmoil can arise, from how easily a person can go from your rock to a stranger. **If I were to do one thing over again, it'd be to leave him before he left me.**

That night was the last time I saw Sean alone. He had a new girlfriend following a week or so of cold silence, which seemed a lot more like gruesome words speaking at the rate of a million per minute. Her name is Courtney. She makes it clear she doesn't like me, but can you blame her? I couldn't make her new boyfriend happy. Now, she has to pick up my slack.

She is petite-a beautiful body, in my opinion. A brief peek at her small frame flipped on the switch inside of me that reminded me why I don't deserve to eat. She is a walking trigger to me. Together, the two are destroying me. They stomp on me, throw me around, hit me and knock me down. I let them. There is not a day I didn't get to hear or see them promoting their happiness together. There is one thing they didn't do, and that's starve me. I did that all on my own. Now, the only time I get to see him is in my dreams. My mind has me held hostage, but that's ok. **At least I'm my own prisoner now, rather than his.**

27
October, 2013
When I Needed You the Most, You Weren't There

It's five-thirty on a Saturday morning, and I'm having five-thirty on a Saturday morning thoughts. You know how when you fail a test or a family member dies, you get this sick pit within the absolute bottom of your stomach that suppresses your appetite to the point where you're not exactly sure when you'll ever be hungry again?   I feel like that all of the time. Maybe that's why I don't eat.

It's October. I like to act like things are going well for me. I try not to look back at pictures of Sean and I, I try to act like the situation has not once bothered me. But it does. When no one is looking, I cry. Hard. I work all of the time, but I'd rather just sleep. I'm so cold, and tired.

I'm working the six-forty five to twelve o'clock shift today, and I'm already dreaming of the warm bed I get to lay in when I get home. That's right, lay in. In my free time I lay in bed, mostly because I'm so tired all of the time. I don't sleep though, because I can't. Even when I do get the opportunity to get plenty of sleep, in between waking up to the sound of my own stomach growling and the anxiety of breakfast in the morning, I'm still exhausted all of the time. I wish I knew why. It's a feeling that won't go away.

They say our worst battles are between what we want and how we feel. I want to eat, but I feel fat. It's that simple. Before I eat breakfast, I weigh myself. Ninety-five pounds and six ounces. My stomach twists into a tight knot when I have to look at the scale and no longer see a former eighty-two pounds. I'd like to think I'm recovered, but with my state of mind, I know I'm not.

I swallow my eighty-calorie yogurt cup and black coffee, only to find myself rushing back to the scale one more time before I hit the road. Ninety-six pounds on the dot. I could throw up. Trying to shake off the feeling of seeing your weight go up is like trying to breathe without any oxygen. It just doesn't work.

I really should have been more aware of how Sean treated other people. It didn't cross my mind once that *that* was going to be how he would end up treating me.

28 November, 2013

A Walk in the Hallways

You know, there's a reason why relationships in high school don't last. It's because we all care too much about the 'what ifs'; we picture ourselves married with children to our high school sweethearts and think about what our lives would be like if we were open to other people throughout the many years we have ahead of us. The what ifs scare us. We get scared and we run away. Maybe from what could've been a huge mistake, and maybe what could've been the best thing that has ever happened to you.

In Sean's situation, I don't find that to be the case. I don't think he realizes how fragile I am both mentally and physically, or cares.

As I walk through the dark hallways of North Valley, I scroll through twitter. My eyes are instantly attracted to a tweet by Sean, and as my stomach drops I try to mentally prepare myself to read it.

"She's everything you never were. #sohappy"

I immediately run to the bathroom. No one understands how easy it truly is to break me. You're not the one who has to go home to a pair of scissors held up to your wrist wondering which decision to make; you can merely resume with your everyday life as if nothing ever happened. You have walls. Walls that aren't even cracked when spite slithers out of your lips and plunge into my mind where it is the most fragile. My walls had been brutally torn down years ago. You can easily pick me apart, without even realizing it, left and right. From here, I find my only option is to pick myself apart.

She's everything you never were. It's one thing to make sure I personally know I wasn't enough for him, but it's another to make sure all 474 of his followers know as well. There's a lot of horrible things you can say to a person, or even just about a person. It's always going to be a tie between that and "she got too skinny, so I left her."

Dear Reader,

Social media is powerful. Words are powerful. Know that with every word you post, especially when directed at someone specifically, you may be inflicting a load of emotions on them. Be careful what you put out there.

29
November
2013

School Lunch

11:58 am

"IT'S NACHO DAY," I hear Zach shout across the room to Tyler. I sigh.

Every day at 12 pm, the bell rings, and all of the normal students rush off to lunch. I, on the other hand, gradually make my way over to the cafeteria, anxious about my pre-established routine.

I get to our table-mine, Avril's and Alisha's spot.

Avril is my best friend. Well, I guess now I should say was. We were once borderline inseparable, until a damper was put on our tight bond the minute I turned from excitingly crazy to physiologically crazy. Funny how that works.

We were like sisters since the second grade. We went from planning what color we would wear every day at school to buying our first bras together, from our first day of high school together to dating boys for the first time. We never had to go through anything alone, that   is, until I got sick.

She wanted to help me, but was smart enough to know there was no chance saving someone who didn't want to be saved. Believe it or not, I was once a really fun person. We were the kind of friends that had trouble calming down from laughing at something in class until the teacher threatened to separate us. We bonded through getting ice cream together, making jokes and laughing until our entire core hurt; it blows me away to think of doing such a thing now.

When Avril and Alisha get laughing, like laughing hard, I really can not comprehend it. I don't understand how someone can just effortlessly laugh like that. I don't remember what it's like to find something funny enough to laugh at, or even something worth genuinely smiling over.

So here, at lunch everyday, I get to be reminded where I went wrong, and what a valuable person I have lost. I get to watch those two laugh and attempt to include me, but we all really know I'm not actually a part of this-and by this, I mean life. Avril isn't the best at expressing her emotions, but I see it in her eyes every time we're here, at that lunch table; we meet eye-to-eye, steamed vegetables and raspberries versus peanut butter sandwich and Oreos, guilt versus happiness, forced smiles versus a genuine laugh. That's where we went wrong, when I didn't have the energy to laugh at her jokes anymore, to smile and laugh and chew and gossip like nothing had ever changed.

Dear Reader,

Yes, sick. Eating disorders and depression are illnesses.

30

November, 2013

My 'Willpower'

I hate myself. My body may struggle to live, but my mind is ready to die. That's what nobody seems to understand. I can't think straight when I'm starving, but the thing is, I thrive from that feeling. It's like this little skinny bitch got into my mind and decided to take over whenever I need to listen or comprehend something important. The feeling of starvation is the one sense of both accomplishment and pride that I can grasp onto every day.

When I tell my parents I'm "getting better," they act as if they believe it. Deep down, I know they don't. If we pretend like nothing's wrong, maybe eventually it won't be.

I am stronger than everyone else because I can control myself. Why does everyone try to get me to eat? They're all just jealous, jealous because their thighs touch while mine don't. They all want me to be fat, just like them.

I have something on all of them, something on everybody. I know how to say no. My eating disorder makes me special. I've never been special before, and now I am; it takes a crazy amount of willpower to deny yourself food. *Hungry and cold. Cold and hungry.* They aren't even feelings anymore, but personality traits. This is who I am: hungry, cold and tired, but strong. I am winning. I'm always winning. It's so great. Like the other day, in school for example:

Holly brought in brownies. She offered them to Amelia, Alisha, Amber, and me. They're homemade, too, and just for the record, I have never seen such a gooey and moist chocolate dream in my entire life. I watch as they all dive into the container. I sit here. I would do anything for one of those brownies, just one. Maybe I'll have just one. No. I could never be able to have "just one." Strong. Stay strong. You're starving, and if you give in, you break. You won't stop until you're full. Who knows when I'll <u>finally</u> be full? After months on months of starving, I'd imagine it would take months on months to become full. I'd never stop eating.

So I won't. If I don't eat, I don't have to worry about not being able to stop. Then I won't be fat. *How do they do it?* How do they just eat in the spur of the moment like that? I can't think back to when I was able to do that... just eat when I'm offered something. I have to plan. Be precise of what I will be allowed and how much of it, because I am strong and won't push my limits.

If I were to push my self imposed limits, I'm pretty sure I'd have to kill myself. There's no way I could live with the hate and frustration I'd have for myself all over again. I may be strong, but I'm not that strong. I can't gain weight. I'll feel the exact way I did when I had to lose the weight. And <u>I will</u> lose it again if it comes down to it. If my thighs ever touch again, I won't be able to forgive myself. Every time I pass a mirror, I feel compelled to stop dead in my tracks. I know the drill. Feet together, eyes on the thighs. I lift up my shirt. Stomach small, could be flatter. Hip bones show, could be more noticeable. Body thin, could be perfect.

Why do I stare only at my body? I can't remember the last time I looked in the mirror and saw my own eyes. I'm not even sure what color they are anymore. No boobs, just collarbones. No butt, just thigh gap. No smile, just cheekbones. No life, just breathing. I'm not even sure which option I like better. Being dead may actually be better than being alive. At least when you're dead, you don't have to feel the pain anymore. Then you're numb and empty, but strong.

This path is so lonely. **I hate being alone.** However, I'm never alone, because at the end of the day, my eating disorder is always there, waiting for me with open arms. It's the one thing I can truly count on. I've learned that I cannot count on people, their words or their promises. I can't count on money. Money won't buy me any sort of happiness. Everyone and everything lets me down in one way or another. Maybe that's why I always go back to anorexia, because it's always there for me. *Always.*

Dear Reader,

I want you to know this comes from a mind that truly was not well. At the time, I believed this with every part of my withering being. However, just because something, or someone, is there for you, doesn't mean that it or they are good for you.

31

December 2014

Good-byes

Sometimes I question myself. I question what is my fault and what isn't. Maybe my life is like this because I stayed with Sean, even when I knew it wasn't right. Maybe it's because I allowed myself to be his temporary girlfriend, his crutch. I'm not sure why I let him, either. Maybe because seeing him was the only time I could ever feel somewhat wanted, like I was almost loved. I craved that love stronger than I craved the feeling of being empty inside.

I always think, "I'm going to bed. I don't want to be awake anymore." By that, I mean that it's the closest thing I can get to death right now. Even when wishing my own ending, I think about other people. I picture my mom, tearing herself apart over my grave, questioning what she could've done differently. Pondering how she failed as a mother. My dad, patting her back gently, comforting her, convincing her that life isn't for everyone, and we all can't push away our inner demons; my brother, holding hands with his girlfriend, coming to a realization that she is now the only primary female in his life, other than mom. I can even see my own dog, sniffing around my room, wondering where I am, as my mom is forced to go in my former sanctuary and drag him out while tears well up in her eyes due to the memory of me. I know I have people that would care if I was gone, but I can't get my own being to care. Starving myself has been the slowest, most painful suicide I can think of. If I deserve to die, I deserve to take the hard way out.

I don't even want to admit it, but I am not satisfied with the way things ended with Sean. I never thought the last time was going to be the last. I didn't think that last goodbye meant goodbye forever. I didn't think he would cut the last string of hope I had left for him right then and there. We lose things without warning; and in my opinion, the most agonizing goodbyes are the ones that were never said, and some of the most painful losses are over someone who's still living. We won't all wake up one day and realize our time is over; death comes without warning, and so do goodbyes. We think there will be more. We think we have forever, when we don't.

He wasn't sure of me the way I was sure of him. I chose him every day, and he couldn't choose me for one of them. He didn't see my love as rare, or even worthy. When you tell the truth, that truth buries itself into a part of your past.   However, lies are different. Every time you tell a lie, it becomes part of your future. In the end, Sean was always lying. That's his future in my eyes, just one massive lie. I thought that if you acted like the world revolved around you than that's all you would end up with, yourself. However, he's with her, and I'm alone.

32

December, 2014

Christmas Time

Getting excited for presents on Christmas is a lot easier when you're a kid. Of course everyone likes getting things, but it's not the same when you know nothing can make you smile anymore. If people can't make me smile, why would presents make me smile? That's right, they don't. I do know for a fact, however, what would make my mom's entire Christmas worthwhile: pumpkin bread. Before my grandma had passed, it was a family tradition for all three of us to bake pumpkin bread together before the holidays. When she did pass, my mom and I carried on the tradition for her. For my entire life, Christmas morning consisted of presents and pumpkin bread.

Eating it.

As I open all of my presents, not a single one can make me sincerely happy. The only bit of joy I got out of Christmas was watching my family open the things I got them. If I can't be happy, I'm at least glad they can be. However, seeing my mom's face as I eat pumpkin bread will be the most rewarding thing I can see this Christmas.

"So," she prods, "are you going to have some pumpkin bread with us?" She look hopeful. Maybe even enough hopeful for the both of us.

"A small piece," I manage to murmur.

"Butter?"

"No thank you." Let's not push it.

As I put the bread to my mouth, I can't even enjoy it. I know it physically tasted good, but mentally all I can taste is the cup of fattening shortening, the cup of real sugar, the whole eggs and the white flour. Everything I've avoided. Each bite becomes harder and harder. This is why all of my days are premeditated, so I don't end up in this position. Not like I haven't contemplated this pumpkin bread for months ahead of time, but maybe I could've assembled a plan to give a few bites to my dog or hide away bits and pieces in my napkin. Instead I'm here, absorbing every last calorie, hating myself for it.

I finish the entire piece of bread in front of my mother. She looks honored. As satisfying as the look was, it wasn't enough to stop me from rushing to the bathroom to step on the scale. Ninety-four point six.

My mind clings to the number. I've gained so much. I miss the summer where I was skinny, eighty pounds skinny. Why hasn't my body stayed at that?

Right, because I'm a fucking pig who eats fifteen grams of fat in one sitting. I don't deserve anything for the rest of this day. Not even my yogurt cup, nothing; so, I kneel in front of my parent's toilet and get ready to taste the pumpkin bread again. This is my comfort zone, where I belong. My eating disorder is my comfort zone.

I stick 2 fingers to the back of my throat. I keep them there. I begin to gag, but I keep them there- that's when the food starts to seep up between my fingers. I keep them there. I start to cry.   Food and tears land in the toilet simultaneously, but I still keep them there. It's like I can feel my grandma is looking down at me, ashamed of who I have become. *This is what I am good at, Grandma. Please don't be mad. This is why I am powerful.* I clean myself up as fast as possible and go downstairs. Here, I will have some water and pretend to eat a couple of carrots at our family dinner. Then, I'll lay in bed for the next 10 hours regretting my decision, waiting for the appropriate time to sleep for the night.

Merry Christmas.

33

January 2014

Rock Bottom

It's one thing to starve yourself, but it's another thing to realize that you are actually doing it. I never *wanted* things to turn out this way. It all started as something that made me feel valued; something I endured throughout my traumatic downfall with Sean, something that furnished me with a deranged, erroneous sense of control. Until over time it spiraled out of my reach, curving into a disease that both controlled and consumed me. I used to do it for him; to be worthy of him, to be perfect for him. He's not even in my life anymore, and I still can't stop.

I struggle to sit in class without my mind wandering away. It seems every time I sit in that cold, unpleasant excuse for a chair, my entire being shivers. My thoughts saunter away into the mental planning of what to eat next, when to eat it, and how long I can get away with avoiding it until I feel as if my heart is about to terminate. I wouldn't eat at all if I didn't feel my heart slow down a little too much here and there. Too risky.

Attempting to hang out with friends is a headache. Not only because everyone knows I bring absolutely no light to the party, but because pretending to be healthy gets too exhausting for me. Acting like I'm not quivering the night away causes conflict between my eating disorder and I; it wants me to shiver, it desires me to be the skinny girl who drops dead in the middle of a social event.

I want help. Vegetables and plain Greek yogurt cups shouldn't have to qualify for my meals anymore.   It's moments like this that have me sprawled out across my bed, hands yanking on my own hair, calling my mom to me as if a wildfire had sparked and had me trapped in my own room without any chance of escaping. As my mother made her way up the stairs, her expression simmering a bit when making notice of my tributary of tears upon my own sheets.

"What's wrong?" she asks.

"Mom, I can't do this anymore. I need help. We all like to think I'm getting better, when we all know that I'm not."

"Morgan, what do you mean... I thought you said you were getting better?"

"I'm not, how can you be so oblivious to that? Normal girls don't bring their own steamed vegetables to family birthday parties. Normal girls don't refuse to go out with their friends because they are too exhausted from lying in bed all day. Normal girls don't sit at the dinner table with their family and refuse to partake in their meals, their conservations and their love for the life they are living. I'm not a normal girl, and at this point, that's all I want to be."

Every time I talk like this to my mom she gives me "the look." "The look" brings me back to being a child, where neither of us saw this coming. To me, it's like saying, "honey, your father and I would never have had you if we had known you'd end up trying to kill yourself." It's not like I saw this coming. Life throws you curve balls, curve balls that you cannot possibly fathom. Life tests your faith in ways that seem so vehemently wrong. People affected by eating disorders are like dominos. When the victim is knocked down, the disease continuously and turbulently takes out everything in front of them.

My mother has disappeared to talk to my dad, and as usual, I expected the same routine: they talk, then talk to me and then expect me to get my shit together. Which never happens. Today was different though. My dad woke me up the next morning, informing me that I had an appointment.

"It's in South Grayburn" he began, "only about an hour and a half away. It's called Willington Behavioral Care, and one of their specialists requested if she could evaluate you. I said yes."

A part of me wants this for myself. I want to regain my health and my life and pick up where I left off before everything in my life collapsed. Yet, another part of me doesn't want them to stop me. I'm afraid that if I gain weight, I'd be right back at square one; and the cycle would just keep repeating. Honestly, I'm probably not even sick enough for any sort of medical attention. I'm too fat to be anorexic. I put shame to all anorexics for not being skinny or sick enough. Who knows, maybe the woman who evaluates me will just end up laughing in my face. I don't deserve any care.

Dear Reader,

Yes, despite how incredibly thin and frail I was I did think this. So much of how we see ourselves in this world is through glasses of our own perception... and too often those glasses are skewed by someone else's words-the media, magazine images of women who have had a computer touch up all the "imperfections", etc. Imperfections are what make us unique, it is part of our beauty.

34

January, 2014

Why Aren't You in School Today, Morgan?

When I arrive at Willington, the first thing they did was have me go into a small bathroom and take all of my clothes off. They gave me a hospital gown to put on. Before I do, I look at myself in the mirror. I am tan, really tan. I see skin peeling off of my stomach due to the dryness of it. My stomach appears to be bloated, yet my rib cage makes quite the noticeable appearance. My legs stand far apart, even when I put them the closest they can be together. My chest is flat, my hair is dull, and my facial expression is lifeless. I take out my phone and take a picture.

Never once in my life did I think I could hate what I saw *that* much. I've experienced bad hair days and pimples, but never before this have I seasoned looking in a mirror and finding myself to be a waste of life. I reluctantly substitute my oversized undergarments for the worn out hospital gown. I slowly make my way out of the bathroom, where the woman who will be evaluating me, Anna, asks me to step on a very thin and futuristic looking scale. She keeps her eyes peeled on a small laptop, where I'm guessing my weight has appeared. She immediately closes the laptop and keeps up with a constant poker face.

"Alright Morgan, change back into your clothes. You and I are going to talk alone for a bit, without your parents."

"Wait," my voice crackling, "what was my weight?"

Anna smiles and gives me the "you know better than to ask me that" look. I slowly turn back around and make my way into the bathroom, where I put all of my clothes back on. Before following Anna into her office, I take one last look at the photo I took of myself in the bathroom mirror. *I sure have changed, haven't I?*

Anna led me into her office. "Take a seat. I am going to ask you a few questions just to get a little background information on you." I hate how she's acting; like I don't know what she is doing or why I am here. "Morgan, what did you eat yesterday?"

I like how she knows that I'll remember every last bite. Good job Anna, you got that part of your job right, and that's knowing anorexic qualities. For a minute, I pondered whether I should lie or not. I don't really have anything to lose, so I might as well just tell her the truth.

"I woke up around seven and ate a Greek yogurt cup."

"What kind of yogurt cup?"

She actually cares about the content?
    "Dannon light & fit. Then, around 12, I had a ½ cup of light vegetable soup, but I didn't eat any of the noodles or anything. Then around 3, I ate an apple. At like 5 I had one of those pre made salads, basically with lettuce, some egg, and some imitation crab meat in it. It came with a Caesar dressing that I threw away."

"Is that everything?" She is typing rapidly as I speak.

"Yes."

"Do you smoke?"

"Yes."

"Drink?"

"Yes."

"How often do you partake in these activities, Morgan?"

"Whenever I get the chance to."

"Why?"

I can feel my body tighten up as I wrap my own hand into a tight fist. The harder I squeeze, the more I find myself telling Anna.

"I don't care about myself or what happens to me. I don't think before I do things. I once did, but it was the same reoccurring thought, every single time, and that is that I don't have anything to lose. I mean, what would I have to lose? My life? That's practically already wasted away as it is. My friends? Who would want to be friends with the girl who can hardly pull herself out of bed? My family? They don't even know me. The only time they truly notice me is when I'm laying in my bed at a loss of words because I've been crying that hard. They mean well, they just don't know the first thing about me. I don't have anything to lose, because I have already lost it all. When I have the opportunity to do something that can be considered dangerous and will easily put my life at risk, I jump on it. Why wouldn't I? Maybe something else can kill me besides myself for a change. Right now, heaven sounds like the one chance I have at happiness. And I'm getting closer to it, every damn day."

Anna types a bit more, than asks if I could leave the room for a moment, as she wanted to speak with my parents. I give them their privacy. I don't exactly know what she will even tell them. "Your daughter is psychotic"? Maybe. At least I'm thinner than her.

Anna's door creaks open as she waves for me to come back in. My mom held a stern yet concerned expression, whereas my dad has his face buried within his hands. As he hears my entrance, he looks up from his own palms to reveal his bright-red face, smothered in tears and despair.

"Morgan," he begins, "We... we had no idea you had been doing this to yourself."

His voice is wobbly and unstable, just like his expression. Throughout my entire life, I have rarely seen my dad hurt. He has always been the man I would look at and think, "that's my strong dad." It's not an easy thing, to keep it together when things are always falling apart. My dad always seemed to do it, but not today, as he looks me in the eyes. He sees the eyes *he* created, then looks down at my body, which can only reveal the monster *I* created.

It's one thing to look at someone with your eyes, and it's another thing to look at someone with your mind. In this moment, I have never felt more connected to my father in my entire life. One look into his eyes can take me back to when he was young and tied up with his alcoholism. He had felt my pain, my addiction; maybe even more than I did. His mouth speaks no words, but his eyes scream, "I want my daughter back."

Anna looks back and forth between my parents and me. It is pretty easy to tell she has done this before, but what is even easier was being able to tell that it's agonizing to watch so many families fall apart due to this disease. It is the kind of pain that can make her skin crawl, yet also determine her to go home at the end of the day to a family she can cherish and be even more grateful for having.

"What kind of help can we get her?" My mother's tone is desperate.

"I'm afraid Morgan has one option, and you came to us, so we are obligated to go through with this option and seek the correct medical attention for Morgan. She is going to be inpatient at our Willington out in Waltham, around 3 or so hours away. She will be living there. I can't tell you a definite amount of time she will be there for. It all depends on how she cooperates and improves in terms of her eating disorder. I'm positive you have heard this before, but Morgan has a very severe case of anorexia nervosa."

Both of my parents' jaws drop. My dad nearly jumps out of his seat, to the point where my mom has to hold him down. Anna set off a bomb, a briskly dispersing bomb that has resulted in nothing but panic and dispute that fills the room more and more with each word that comes from her mouth.

"We can't make her an outpatient here? We can't work something out so she can live with us?" Again, my dad's voice shakes beyond both his control and liking.

"Morgan's case is life-threatening. Her weight is currently at 93 lbs., and at her lowest weight of 82 lbs., she was easily a pound or two away from unavoidable death. Nothing against you or your daughter, but she cannot be trusted in the state of mind she is in. She is in need of the best medical attention we have, and that's in Waltham. She needs to live there and focus on the root of her own eating disorder. She has to take charge. She can't do any of that here, especially while living at home. She leaves in two hours."

"Two hours?!" My parents voices are in sync.

"But Snoball..." I begin.

The Snoball is a winter formal my school holds every year. I have plans to go with a guy that I'm sort of friends with in my grade, Cody. It is Saturday. If I left today, there is no way I would make it to Snoball.

"She already has her dress, shoes, and a date...is there any way she can go next Monday instead?" I can tell my dad is thinking of my happiness, as if it isn't already non-existent. Anna sighs. She repetitively looks around the room for a minute or two before she came up with a compromise.

"Okay," she says, "Here's the deal. You have to watch over Morgan. If she loses a single ounce of weight, she's not going to Snoball. Be back here at 8 a.m. next Monday morning, and have all of her things packed. We will evaluate her one more time, then send you all on your way to Waltham."

Everything is now set in stone.

35

January, 2014

Snoball

When you put your dress on, it's supposed to complete the puzzle, right? It's supposed to complement the tight and tedious curls in your hair, along with the meticulous layer of eye shadow that makes your dark eyes pop, drawing attention from the eyes of your envious classmates, right? Wrong.

As I stare at my lethargic reflection in the mirror, I see nothing but dullness. I'm pretty sure everyone else will see that too. When I arrive to take pictures, Cody has shown little to no emotion towards me. As the other girls smile for pictures, I can only curve my lips; even that took a lot out of me. Even if I wanted to I couldn't blend in with everyone else. I know I won't be able to dance much, but for what I can do, I am excited for the calories I will burn.

The dance itself isn't fun. When all the normal people get lasagna, I get salad. When all the normal people dance, I sit. When all the normal people went to party the night away afterwards, I went home to sleep. There isn't much to tell about my Snoball experience, because it turned out to be like every other day for me-lifeless, and struggling to pretend I'm not.

36

February, 2014

Is This Goodbye or Hello?

When my parents and I arrive in North Hampton, Anna is ready for me. We proceed with the same routine: the weigh-in, the questions, and, of course, the stress and attention drawn to my weight- which dropped from my last visit. How I got away with that, I really don't know.

Anna immediately reached residential care out in Waltham. I can't help but agonize over the thought that something could go wrong, skyrocketing my anxiety with every minute. After a solid five minutes, Anna's eyes made contact with mine.

"They are expecting you in two hours. Good luck, Morgan." Here we go, we are on our way.

I'm not even depressed or scared anymore, I'm just kind of numb. I can't tell if that's a beautiful thing, or a horribly despairing type of thing. Everything was once so heart-rending for me, but now I just walk around with this anesthetic look on my face. I didn't expect to adjust to this kind of pain, but I did. How does it make sense, that my mind is really spinning, but I feel nothing? It's a radiant type of silence, and paralyzing the pain may just excruciate it even more when it finally hits.

In Waltham, the first thing I had to do was say goodbye to my parents. They are horrified, and I know that, so I have to at least try and be appalled with them. Maybe one day I can feel the emotion I've been pretending to have. I have to give my phone up, as well. The last text I got was from Avril.

She knew where I was physically headed, but she didn't know where I am headed mentally. I think that's what scares her. She is the one who gave me a text to remember before giving up my phone. I could've thought about the social media, the anorexic girls I follow on Instagram- the skinny girls and the models and the pro ana websites, but what stuck with me before giving that toxic piece of plastic away was Avril.

"I'm scared for you. I mean it Morgan, don't leave there until you trust yourself again."

That is what was stuck in my head as I prepare myself for the routine of this place. They stick you in this one room here the majority of the time. It's a living room type setting, maybe to make you feel like you're at home, but at home, no one checks your pee before you are allowed to flush. The other patients here are just like me, monotonous and dejected. I mean, you know what they say, what doesn't kill you only makes you wish that it did. Or at least that is the version that resonates with me. The girl sitting next to me hasn't said a word. Come to think of it, none of them actually have. Maybe I'll lighten the mood.

"...Am I the only one here who thinks it's sketchy that the counselors have to look at our shit before we flush it?"

A dull roar of laughter disperses across the room, then one of the quiet girls finally speaks up.

"Right! What if it's a guy counselor...what if we're on our periods?!"

I sigh to myself. "You act like any of us actually get our periods."

"Very true....I'm Leah, by the way."

"I'm Morgan."

Leah. Her eyes sink into her face as she talks. Her sarcastic tone and light-hearted manner suggests to me that she was once a lively girl. It's a shame, because I look at her now and can only see her disease.

Our counselor for the night, Sarah, emerges from her desk. "Alright guys, we're going to head down to dinner."

We gathered together like a group of kindergarteners, walking single file together to take a bathroom break. This isn't kindergarten though and this isn't a bathroom break, this is the reality of an eating disorder. We walk down the hallway to a kitchen-like setting.

The section of this part of treatment is merely one hallway. At the end of it is my room, followed by the rest of the adult rooms. I got roomed with an adult, only because I am 18 and that's all there was available. However, I receive treatment with the adolescents. Along the way down the hall, there are several rooms for the rest of the inpatient adolescents. There are two kitchens, one for inpatients and one for outpatients, who only came from 8 to 5 on weekdays. At the opposite end of the hallway is the school room, where we all attend "school" from 2 to 4 every weekday so we don't have to repeat a grade and fall behind. This is to give us all a fair and equal chance to be normal people once again. Across from that is our living room, where we all cling together and hang around like the life is being sucked out of us at a consistent rate per minute.

When we walk into the "kitchen," we all take our seats with quite a bit of hesitancy. Sarah and one other counselor, Carly, finishes the last bits and pieces of our meals.   As they rapidly look over each individual's meal plan, both counselors go back and forth between us and the counter, matching the correct meal with the correct individual.

Carly places my meal in front of me: it is a sandwich, with what appears to be whole wheat bread-not the 35 calorie kind. In between the two slices of bread are two thick layers of both peanut butter and jelly, I'm guessing two tablespoons of each. On the side, there is a handful of green beans, I'd say around a half cup of cottage cheese and a glass of milk. To estimate, this meal had to be around 500-600 calories; this is more than I would be usually having throughout an entire day.

I've taken a lot of things for granted in my life, but I never thought twice about appreciating being able to eat normally. I never once thought I would struggle with such a thing. Here I am, looking at my day's worth of food in one sitting, trying to keep my face from thawing and my heart from pulsating. I can't play with fire and not expect to get burned.

I eat my meal, all of it. Slowly but surely, I ate. Carly looks over at Hannah and tells her to stop using "behaviors." Hannah stops pushing her food around to make it look like less was there. Diana sticks a glob of peanut butter under the table. She's the girl with the scars that she stares at every time she looks down to eat. Leah keeps kicking her feet and wiggling around. She doesn't finish her milk for a very long time, until she is threatened with a protein shake.

How is being surrounded by the poison supposed to take it away? *Maybe it's because the poison is so relatable that it may just motivate me to get better*. Stupid doctors, don't they realize that when you're enclosed by the triggers they only get worse?

37

February, 2014

How Could I Not Fall in Love With the Pain?

Tonight is our first group therapy. Tia, one of the younger counselors, is holding it this evening. She gathers all of us together in our little living room and announces group is starting.

"Okay guys, tonight's group will be discussing feelings. Feelings that may have contributed to your eating disorder, maybe feelings that take away from it. We're going to go in a circle. Will, you start."

"Alone."

"Elaborate, Will."

Will hesitates.

"Hannah?"

"Frustrating," Hannah mumbles.

"Why is that, Hannah?"

"It's infuriating that all we want are these flat stomachs and thin legs that we can not get, because people like you won't let us."

"Thank you," Tia acknowledges. "Thank you both for sharing. What about you Morgan, what's a feeling, and   why?"

It is finally time for me to speak up.

"Sneaky. Controlling an eating disorder is like controlling a car." All heads are suddenly directed towards me. I continue talking. "You have to make your moves quick. You have to think fast because if you take one wrong turn, your life is gone forever. That's what it feels like, when you're in your kitchen at three in the morning practically eating the core of your apple to keep your own heart from stopping."

Everyone gazes at me as if they are in shock that the new girl has more than one word to say. To be honest, I am a little surprised as well. Tia smiles at me.

38

February, 2014

Misconceptions

"David, we are getting married," I hear Molly yell as the outpatients came to treatment, bright and early for breakfast.

The outpatients only come Monday through Friday, from breakfast to afternoon snack. Molly is an outpatient who lit up a room. Well, made a room dim, I should say. No one here has enough spirit in them to actually lighten a room up. David is one of the two guys here at treatment. Before coming here, I hadn't ever heard of a guy with an eating disorder. It's a big myth, society seems to create, that girls are the only sex under the pressure to be perfect.

Another myth I have recognized about eating disorders is that not everyone that suffers from one is freakishly underweight. Take Mary, for example. Mary is one of the nicest people here at treatment. She is in most of my group therapy sessions, and what isn't so stereotypical about her is that she is actually overweight. People with eating disorders come in all shapes and sizes, I guess there really isn't a certain weight you must be to be considered sick. Mary has confessed to me that she has trouble with cycles of binging and purging, followed by   starvation episodes.

Everyone here has something unique about them when it comes to their eating disorder. So far, that is the only eye opening thing I have experienced about treatment. You don't have to be a girl with a thigh gap to have an eating disorder, because here, despite our weight or gender, we all suffer the same.

39

February, 2014

A Method to the Madness

"Ladies! Weights and vitals!"

Those are the words that every inpatient at Willington forebodes. Why? Here, at Willington, those words mean "it's six in the morning, get up, we need to weigh you but keep that number a secret and then make sure your vitals are stable and force you to drink Gatorade afterwards if you don't meet our standards of healthy." After we get our weights and vitals done, only on Mondays, we get blood taken as well. Typical teenager activities.

This place is stupid. I'm pretty sure the only thing helpful I've learned here is how to knit. Hannah taught Leah, Will and me the other night. Leah and I have become fairly close. We talk about waking up in the middle of the night to do sit ups and how we chose peanut butter over Nutella to go with our pretzels because we know Nutella has a higher sugar content. We giggle together in joy when Leah brought up how the minute we leave this place, we will be the ones in control again. Together, we have the power to kill ourselves in a mental hospital, until we are *forced* to take things seriously.

There has been corruption throughout Willington today. Apparently, we are being brought to a memorial service.

"Who's memorial are we going to?"

Hannah glares at me, then pulls herself in closer towards my ear.   "It's Kelly's memorial."

"Who's Kelly?" The entire group look at me like I had spontaneously grew another head.

"You don't know who Kelly is?" I had never heard Olivia talk until today. She usually just cries when she has to eat red apples instead of green.

"Of course she doesn't know who Kelly is," Will pointed out, "She got here like five days ago. Kelly lived in residential with us, and when she didn't eat for three days, she got moved to Velcott."

"Velcott?"

"Yeah, Velcott. It's the floor under us. It's even more restrictive than us, in weird ways, like not wearing makeup and stuff. Which is hard to believe. You get on feeding tubes there."

"So why are we going to a memorial for this girl..?"

Will looks back to make sure Carly isn't looking.

"Kelly passed away."

It never really hits you how deadly this disease is until you witness people lose their lives over it, practically right in front of you. I don't think I want to die anymore. If people make it out of this place alive, why can't I? I wonder what contributed to Kelly's disease. I wonder if it was a boy, or a self-image issue, the desire to be perfect or all of the above.

I look up from Will's eyes and stare aimlessly at the wall. The one thing that taunts me about this room they throw us in is the walls. There's a series of sides that run horizontally across it. It's song lyrics, a Jessie J song to be exact, that say:

I stare at my reflection in the mirror

Why am I doing this   to myself?

Losing my mind on a tiny error,

I nearly left the real me on the shelf.

Losing my mind on a tiny error. I look down at the gap between my legs. Would it really define me if that space isn't there? Or the perceptible decline in the fat around my hips. Is that really what I need to lose to get someone I love to take note of my existence?   *Shake these thoughts, Morgan. Your eating disorder can't function with this type of thinking.*

I peek over at Olivia. Whenever Leah, Will, Hannah and I are talking or laughing, I always notice her off in the distance, isolating herself more than I thought *even I* ever could.

"Hey Olivia," I probe.

Olivia looks up at me with her big, watery eyes. They are too big for her fragile face.

"Would you want me to teach you to knit? Hannah taught me and it's really relaxing, I think you'd like it."   I can't manage to get a smile out of her, but she nods her head yes; that's all I need.

40

February, 2014

A Reason to Smile

So far, I've been at treatment for about two weeks. I've eaten everything that has been put in front of me...minus the spinach incident. I won't talk about the spinach incident. I'm not even sure why I eat everything. I think it's because you can't necessarily win here. If you don't eat, you get a nutrition shake. If you don't drink your nutrition shake, your meal plan gets bumped up. If you don't eat your new meal plan, you get put on a feeding tube. If you rip that feeding tube out, your heart fails.

In the long run, I'm not going to win here. I realize that the moment I found out Kelly had passed. I can't avoid food anymore. It's everywhere. Food is social. *Don't you want to get pizza with your friends, Morgan?* Food is fun. *Don't you want to bake pumpkin bread with your mom, Morgan?* Food is lively. *Don't you want to live, Morgan?* Food is vital.

41

February, 2014

Reality Hits

I've been teaching Olivia how to knit every night since I've offered to show her. During an activity involving stress, she mentions to the group that she works at a grocery store. I do as well, so I thought maybe I could bring that up during our knitting session.

"Did you know I work at a grocery store, too?"

Olivia hesitates. "Do you really?"

"Yes! Do you like working at one?"

"Well, no. It's kind of triggering."

"Are you referring to the weight loss magazines that we're forced to stare at when we have to wait in front of our register for customers?"

Olivia looks surprised. "Yeah..how'd you know?"

"Look around, Olivia. We're all here with the same problem, all sharing the same mind-set. But I had a thought I'd like to share with you."

"What's that?"

"You and I clearly know a lot about calories in versus calories out, right?"

"Right."

"So when we see these magazines, with these gorgeous woman with photo shopped bodies, claiming they lost thirty pounds in three weeks the *right* way, does that seem realistic to you?"

"I mean...not really.."

"Right. I don't even think I lost that much in that little time and I'm anorexic!!!!"

Olivia's lip curves a bit.

"So my point is," I continue, "If an anorexic girl doesn't even lose thirty pounds in three weeks, why should anyone believe that a woman on the cover of a magazine did? And in a *healthy* way? We are here for treatment, those magazines are intended to appeal to middle-class mothers that want to slim down about thirty to forty unnecessary pounds and are too lazy to actually do it. They're looking for an easy way out. Those magazines are unrealistic, and not for us."

Her slightly curved lips form into a genuine smile, one I haven't seen before, and I'm sure a lot of other people haven't either.

42

February, 2014

A Letter to Me

Today in treatment, we have to write a letter to ourselves, that we will be opening three months from now. I can't imagine what my life will be like in three days, never mind three months. We are given 15 minutes to write this letter, and as soon as my pencil presses to the paper, my mind doesn't rest.

Carly, my favorite counselor, immediately turns her head towards me as our time to write has come to an end. "Morgan, do you want to share your letter?" My eyes meet Carly's, transfixed on the thought of expressing my most profound thoughts and desires to a group of people nearly as fragile as me.

Feb 26th, 2014

Dear Future Morgan,

      I hope you're doing much better than you were three months ago. I'm sure you haven't forgotten this but I'm going to remind you anyway: this place sucks. Please, please don't ever take your home (or your health!) for granted because the minute it's taken away from you, you'll be crying yourself to sleep at night willing to do anything to be in your own bed, in your own home, making your own decisions once again. I beg you, never go back to your old ways. I guarantee you'll end up right here. I hope you take care of your body now. I hope you don't starve or deprive or harm it in anyway anymore. I've learned you can't destroy yourself to victory. It doesn't work like that. I hope you put your energy into something bigger than merely your weight now. I hope you're being productive and making a difference, rather than devoting your entire life to something as insignificant as a number. You deserve to be at peace with yourself. I hope by the time you're reading this you will remember what it's like to eat something without contemplating it for hours. I hope you're stronger than your eating disorder. It isn't selfish to love and respect yourself. You have to spread love instead of being afraid of it. Killing yourself is getting you nowhere, so stop seeing yourself through the eyes of the people who never once valued you. The most important relationship you will ever have is with yourself, so make it a healthy one.

-*The Old You*

43

March, 2014

Discharged

After about a month of inpatient treatment, I was discharged. If you think that isn't a long enough time to change a person, you're right. The following three years after are what really, really changed me.

Weigh-ins follow my discharge. I am not allowed to see the numbers, and I cry almost every time. After revolving your life around numbers for so long, you become sure that is what defines you. It's not. I soon was able to figure out that my weight had been consistently rising. Once I was around 105 lbs., I was convinced that this is going to be my healthy weight. It wasn't.

When I went back to school, people congratulated me. People question me. People think I can now go out for ice cream and love life again. People think that's how recovery goes. They are wrong. The small changes, over long periods of time, turn out to be the foundation of recovery.

There are points where I would contemplate suicide every time something goes wrong. Every single time I feel the tiniest pinch of pain, I become terrified of feeling it the way I used to and immediately wish life ended however many pounds ago. I live in fear, in fear of that negative feeling progressing again and shattering me. I would rather die than barely live again. I soon learn that life is about challenges; you're supposed to face them, instead of run away from them. They'll make you stronger in the long run. Everything you do becomes a lesson.

I spend so much time turning beautiful memories into sour ones. I'll think about them and get sad, because they couldn't happen again. Even if I didn't lose the person I was hurting over, those memories still wouldn't be able to happen again. You can't smile for the exact same reason in the exact same moment a second time. There are things you simply cannot relive and it's a difficult thing to accept and grasp onto, but you have to come to be okay with that. I'm learning to live for the present.

Recovery comes in bursts.

Tonight, only two months out of treatment, when I hugged my mom goodnight, my grasp was much tighter than it used to me.

It wasn't a pity hug or a meaningless goodnight like it used to be.

It was a "thanks for living this day here with me, I can't wait to live the next one with you" kind of hug.

Recovery comes in realizations.

I eventually begin to put as much energy into repelling my eating disorder as I did into feeding it.

It is hard to let go of my eating disorder when I felt like it was the only thing that gave me a purpose. Questioning it is like questioning myself because it consumed and altered that much of me. I realize hunger and power are not linked; self-respect and power are.

Recovery comes with moving on

The prime piece of the puzzle to health is to let go of what brought me down in the first place. It's arduous to accept an apology you never received. I once solely existed in what I thought was the purity of love, before the revelation of the nature of its ambiguity. At first, I wished for Sean to live with a ghost for the rest of his existence, the ghost of the girl who was merely a few pounds away from her deathbed. I wanted her to follow him around, whispering the daunting words he once submerged into my mind with too many destructive intentions that did not possess a single pure nature to restore the damage. Refusing to let go of anger is like running in front of a car and expecting the driver to be the one plowed over in the middle of the road. It's a waste, and for the longest time, I couldn't help but feel that way at the sound of his name. He was the wrong person for me, and that is obvious to the point where it practically jumps out at me and hits me in the face whenever the most subjective part of me has the tiniest urge to miss him. It's insane. It's insane to think that if I would love the wrong person so passionately, imagine how much I could love the right one.

I don't want any of those things for him anymore. All I want out of him is to grow from his past. I want him to feel for a girl the way I felt about him, and treat her as an equal. We say a lot of things in April that we might not mean in May. Words may last forever, but the meaning behind them has no definite consistency. That's why we should be careful about what we say, because those words will never go away.

I no longer look for him in everyone else I meet. I've come to the conclusion that love isn't black or white. Love is grey. It can be viewed as so evil and haunting, yet so precious and valued all at the same time. Love can suspend time and has no depth. Love has a way of alternating many variables, just like the color grey has a way of alternating many other colors. Love itself never fails.

Over time, I am becoming healthy. My eyes that were once such a lifeless pit now light up and glisten with the simple curve of my lips. My lips can speak the truth and make someone's day with a genuine compliment. The lips that can kiss, kiss passionately with both self respect and freedom. The lips that don't quiver when I talk or crack when I fake a smile. I can look at someone and hear what they're saying instead of merely burying their words deep within me and concentrating on nothing but my disease. Things don't go right through me anymore; I don't have to feel so serious all of the time and break down my own walls just to get a laugh out.

I have life inside of me instead of a demon consuming every physical and mental aspect of me with every minute. I've come to flourish into someone who is patient with herself. My life isn't on hold for my eating disorder anymore. I have a lot more to look forward to than harming myself. Watching my body grow wasn't comfortable at first, but that doesn't even compare to how valuable it is to look in the mirror and finally be able to see life in my own eyes.

It can be rare, for people to grow from the mistakes they've made rather than regret them. I don't believe in regrets; I believe that everything happens for a reason. Those reasons are meant to mold you into the person you are, rather than tear you down and become something that hangs over you in remorse every day of your life.

Although I have moved on, I'll never be able to forget him making me feel like I had to apologize for being the person I was. It was torture loving him; *it's the kind of somber suffocation you get addicted to.*

January, 2017

Down the Road: An Epilogue

It's amazing that three years ago I would've never even been able to fathom myself being the person I am today. I am 130 lbs, which is a healthy, sustainable weight for my body. I've eased myself into both intuitively eating and exercising.

Three years ago I would only exercise because I hated my body, trying to burn whatever calories my fragile body was able to handle. I now am able to listen to my body, exercising when appropriate because I am passionate about seeing myself becoming physically and mentally stronger with each day that passes. The day upon which this was realized was a day that changed my life forever.

I'm no longer about temporary things: temporary people, temporary feelings, or a temporary state of mind. I'm about consistency and determination. I've learned that if you want results you've never had, you have to do things you've never done before. The friendships I had lost in the midst of my eating disorder are the ones I gained back when I gained back my weight.

I no longer shut anyone out. I gained back the energy to maintain, and even create, balanced and stable friendships, but more importantly, the person I once was I now see again in the mirror- only stronger.

When I look back upon my eating disorder I see nothing other than empty years. The fifty pounds I was missing was my life. That weight was cake on my birthday, turkey on Thanksgiving, and cookies on Christmas. That weight was sleeping through the night. It wasn't waking up to extreme hunger pangs or enduring an anxiety attack over having to eat breakfast in the morning. My happiness used to be determined by measurements; now it's insistent on moments.

In the three years that has passed I often get asked about what factors contributed to my eating disorder. *Was social media triggering you...? Did Instagram have an impact on my self-esteem...?* Looking back now, I truly believe the "feed" did negatively factor into the person I saw each and every day. I found myself drawn to an absurd amount of weight loss "thinspo" accounts. These accounts plastered my news feed daily by flaunting starving bodies that I thought I desired at the time. In addition to the tempting skeletons, were many fad diets or some ludicrous sit up challenge that in all reality would never actually work. I once thrived off these posts, but soon realized how they were affecting me. You can't control what people post, but you can control whom you follow and the impact it has on your life.

In addition to social media, I now know and understand that society can impact how people view their bodies. It took me the longest time to realize that the majority of today's models are unhealthy. Even when I'm online shopping and I see the measurements of the model on the side, I shake my head. Typically, it's a really tall height and some ridiculously unreasonable measurements. Followed by these measurements, the site reveals that the model is wearing a size small. So many people look at those statistics and think that's where they should be, and I was one of them for far too long. One of the most manipulating things society can do for anyone's body image is teach them models are supposed to be 5'11" and weigh as much as someone who's healthy and 5'4".

Throughout my lost years, I let someone who was no longer in my life continue to hurt me. I no longer allow anyone to dictate the person I see in the mirror. It's okay to miss someone, but it's not ok to give them the power to endlessly tear you down. If someone I care about no longer wishes to be a part of my life, the best thing I can do for myself is accept it and move on. I am no one's puppet; I've cut ties with toxic people.

Another thing I've learned is that everyone's body is unique. We all have different bodies, different heights, different metabolisms, and different physical and mental needs. I now live comfortably in my body, despite my goals. My aspiration now is to be the best version of myself, and for the first time in my life just enjoy the process.

Now, I don't have to cherish the process alone. I once merely left my body at someone's doorstep, yet never left my soul in the hands of someone who cares.

I am more than just a body.

Dedications

This book is dedicated to my loving family and friends, and anyone and everyone who has helped or supported me along my journey.

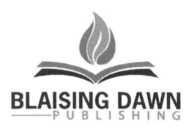

www.blaisingdawn.com

Blaising Dawn Publishing was created with the belief that each of us has a story to tell, but often times find it difficult knowing how to share our story with the world. With the deepest passion for health, wellness & living a balanced life, Scott & Shera Dawn continue their quest by helping each of you share your message.

More from Blaising Dawn Publishing:

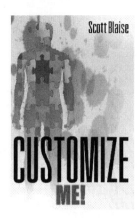

Scott Blaise

CUSTOMIZE ME!